Before the 'Crop' Comes Out

Before the 'Crop' Comes Out

8 essentials to consider before disciplining your horse

SANDI BELL

Before the 'Crop' Comes Out : 8 essentials to consider before disciplining your horse
Sandi Bell

ISBN: 978-1-936214-53-2
Library of Congress Control Number: 2012930357

©2012 Sandi Bell
All Rights Reserved.

Illustrations © and Interior Design by April Ollig Milne – Equestrian Impressions
Interior Photographs by courtesy of Sandi Bell
Cover Photo © by Somogyvari/Istock photo
Cover Design © by Nancy Cleary and Sandi Bell
Contributor & Research by Linda Purves
Editing by Linda Purves & Mike Bell

All rights reserved. No part of this book may be reproduced or transmitted in any manner whatsoever without written permission except in the case of brief quotations embodied in critical articles and reviews. All inquiries should be addressed to Heart and Soul Equine Publications, P.O. Box 1338 Santa Clara, CA 95052. www.heartandsoulequine.com.

The information in this book is true and complete to the best of our knowledge. All recommendations are made without guarantee on the part of the author or publisher. The author and publisher disclaim any liability in connection with the use of this information

Heart and Soul Publications books may be purchased in bulk at special discounts for sales promotions, corporate gifts, fund-raising, or educational purposes. For details contact Heart and Soul Equine Publications, P.O. Box 1338 Santa Clara, CA 95052. www.heartandsoulequine.com.

All Trademarks belong to their respective owners.

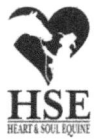

Published by Heart & Soul Equine Publications, Imprint of Wyatt-MacKenzie
www.heartandsoulequine.com

*To both my Mom and Dad, your love for animals
has been woven into my DNA ...*

*and to my horse Grace, my equine soul mate,
you are 'My Saving Grace,' and a reflection of all that is good.*

Acknowledgements

Along with any creative idea come choices on how to best express it. It's a process that takes time. I have been blessed with true encouragement while writing this book. Many, who may or may not have known it, bolstered me along the way.

First, I would like to express my thanks to Linda Kalamasz. Meeting you several years ago began a turning point for me that re-awakened my passion and started me on this amazing journey of discovery. Your love and compassion for horses, your intuitive care, respect and understanding of these noble creatures as individuals is beautiful and rare. You taught me the value of being a horse's advocate. For your inspiration and insight I am eternally grateful.

To Lisa Orrell for helping me launch this book and Nancy Cleary for helping me get it published, my sincere thanks.

To my long time friend April Milne, your creative ability and horsewoman know-how have been a blessing to me. Thank you for your time and talent in helping me illustrate this book and bring it to life. You are a special lady and I could not have had a better partner.

Another blessing has been the love and support of my friend Cyndi Perry. Your willingness to be a part of any endeavor of mine, at a moment's notice, is truly God's love in action. Putting me first and being thoughtful is routine for you. You are such a wonderful lady and I am truly grateful to have met you and to know you. You are my 'barn angel.'

And to Jacki Cramer, whose courage in life I admire, I am pleased to call you my friend. I will always appreciate your clear, intuitive and intelligent guidance in refining the direction and purpose of this project. You are amazing.

And last but not least, to my husband, Mike Bell. You have done nothing but support me in every endeavor I have ever pursued. It is not only your daily encouragement that helps me to believe in myself and to make something like this happen, but your intelligence and strong ability to persevere in spite of difficult situations that I admire and strive to emulate. You are more loved than you know.

Preface

If someone had asked me a year ago if I thought I would write a book, I might have answered: "maybe someday." Although writing a book was on my bucket list, like so many things it was buried beneath the busy-ness of my life until a true purpose came to light.

Horses offer us so much more than recreation or sport; they can enhance and enrich our lives and our understanding of ourselves. They are divine creatures, perfectly created, with real needs and feelings not unlike our own, that without understanding, we can overlook and neglect. We can so easily misinterpret a horse's behavior that we often discipline them for things beyond their control, unknowingly making the situation worse. When they're in pain or discomfort, they can't use words to make us understand. That is why I wanted to write this book, to speak on their behalf.

I also wrote this book to encourage horse owners. This is information that I hope will help you bring the best out of both you and your horse, so don't give up. Who knows? You might be in for something special.

We all have visions of who we are and what we want out of our lives, then suddenly life takes an unexpected turn and we find ourselves somewhere we never expected to be. The stages in life when you lose equilibrium, to me, are the best times for growth. It is during these difficult times when I have always learned the most about myself, and my faith; when I realize deeply that I just need to let go, that by trusting everything is 'as it should be,' one can keep moving.

This past year has been a journey that I would not trade for the world. My eyes have been opened to new information, new possibilities and new paths. By grace, I have been able bring my passion to light on these pages during one of the most trying years of my life. For that I am deeply grateful.

Table of Contents

Acknowledgments vii

Preface ix

Introduction 1

**Chapter 1   Understanding Your Horse's Legs
               and Good Basic Shoeing** 7
• Hoof and Leg Function • Is Your Horse a Sound, Fully Functioning Horse?
• Checking for Lameness • Other Contributing Factors to Lameness • Basic Shoeing
• Basic Shoeing Check • Owner Responsibilities • Grace's Story

Chapter 2   Why Chiropractic and Massage 19
• What is Equine Chiropractic? • Behavioral Issues Connected to Subluxation
• Finding Hidden Pain • Simple Chiropractic Back Check • Checking for Muscle
Tension • Maintaining a Pain and Tension Free Body • Tension Remedies
• Keeping It All Together • An Ounce of Prevention • Grace's Story • Sound
Asleep in the Arena

Chapter 3   Understanding Saddle Fitting Basics 27
• Grace's Story • Why Bother? • Ill-fitting Saddle Behavior • What Lies Under
Our Saddles? • Basic Parts of the Saddle • How to Check the Saddle Itself
• Things to Look For Before Fitting • Check List for Good Basic Fit • Rider Fit
• Final Notes on Fitting

Chapter 4   Bit Choice and Bit Resistance 41
• Grace's Story • What Might Be Wrong With Our Bit Choice? • Snaffle Bit verses
Curb Bit: What's the difference? • Bit Mouthpieces • Common Bit Resistance
Issues • Understanding the Mouth • Bit Width Sizing • Common Misconceptions
and Next Steps • A Change in the Industry

Chapter 5   Nutrition Basics and Dental Awareness 51
• Grace's Feeding Story • Looking At The Big Picture • The Natural Digestive Design • Nutritional Things to Keep in Mind • Feed Basics • Reading Feed Tags • What Is In Your Horse's Diet? • Choosing the Right Feed for Your Horse • Feeding Guidelines • What Is the Right Amount Food? • Measuring Your Horse's Weight with a Tape • Horse Body Condition Scoring • Feed Rations and Your Horse's Level of Activity • Weight Management • Malnutrition and Sugar Behavioral Issues • Routine Dental Care – A Must! • Grace's Dental Story

Chapter 6   Conditioning and Stretching 63
• Grace's Story • The Warm Up • Simple Stretches • Preparing and Judging the Correct Amount of Exercise • The Boredom Factor • Be Fair • Don't Forget the Cool Down • Preventing Injury • The Weekend Trail Ride • The Equine Athlete

Chapter 7   Grooming and Good Husbandry 69
• Our Story • Reasons for Grooming • Grooming Essentials • A Grooming Routine • Horse Husbandry Considerations • Care with Respect

**Chapter 8   Understanding Who You Are as a Rider
               and Choosing a Mentor** 77
• Who We Are as Riders • Leaving Your Problems Behind • Have Clear Intentions for Your Ride • Rider Fitness – A Big Deal! • Choosing a Mentor • Follow Your Heart • Wrapping It Up • My Wish for Every Horse and Rider

Resources 85

Bibliography 87

Introduction

I wrote this book for all of the horses in our lives.

Most folks begin their stories by telling of how young they were when they first got involved with horses and of all the twists and turns they have taken on their 'horsey' journey from that point forward. My own story could be told that way, but what I really want to share with you is a true story that sent me off on a new journey. My story starts when I met a horse named Dove.

I was attending a week long riding instruction certification program in a nearby town. I was excited to start what I was anticipating to be a week of fun and intense study, ready to begin another new chapter in my life with horses. The first day began with us, seven ladies and one gentleman, getting acquainted as a group. I, along with the other attendees, had signed up to spend the entire week honing my teaching skills, which was to include riding several different horses each day. Unbeknownst to me, spending time with the others and learning together was to become only part of an experience that changed my life forever.

After a brief round table introduction, our group leaders encouraged us to voice our wishes and desires for the certification, along with sharing our horsey backgrounds, as part of the meet and greet. After this discussion was finished, we were taken outside to locate our new partners for the day. I was introduced to Dove. A lot of time was wasted that first morning searching for tack and other miscellaneous items each individual horse needed. It quickly became obvious that there would be virtually no time to bond with the horses. We were to "get 'em ready, hop on, and get riding," and left with little time to groom properly. With the little time I had, I noticed that Dove was particularly bothered when I ran the brush along his back. Each time I did so, he would swing his head around as if to say "ouch!" Though there was a definite rush to get ready, I felt compelled to tell one of the leaders about Dove's issue. To my surprise, my concern was instantly dismissed due to the program's pressing time line. I reluctantly saddled and bridled the poor animal and proceeded to follow instructions, a deep feeling of discomfort lingering in my soul.

The entire time I was on Dove's back I was keenly aware that he was hurting. His pain was evident with every step he took.

When the long eight hour day of riding was finally complete we un-tacked our horses. Once again, only a few moments remained to do a quick groom before putting the horses back in their stalls. Dove was still hurting. I would have taken the time to address his discomfort, but we apparently had a more pressing engagement—we were to meet with the group for a rundown of the next day's activities.

The next morning, we quickly got back into clinic mentality. We were assigned our horses for the day and low and behold, I got Dove. I rechecked my observations from the previous day and found the same reaction in Dove's back as I carefully brushed it. This time I approached the other leader to tell her of my discovery, which led to a minor victory when she acknowledged that the horse did have some irritation. The instructor decided that he should be "rested" for the day. Finally, I could relax on a different horse.

Wednesday arrived and the morning's event was to be an hour and half's trail ride. I must have become a source of irritation, or a pain in the neck, where Dove was concerned, as I had been assigned a different horse for the day. We were split into two groups, each group accompanied by one of the clinic leaders. My group left first. The trail ride took us up gradual hillsides, with only a few minor moments of steeper terrain. It was a smooth ride with no disasters. When we got back, it was the second group's turn to ride. I remember the feeling I got in the pit of my stomach once again as I realized another woman rider was paired with poor Dove for the trail ride. He was tacked, ready to leave with the other group. I watched them set out for the steady climb that I knew was at the beginning of the trail, I could feel my empathy increase and my heart broke for him as I watched him walk off.

Our leader kept us busy for the next hour and a half, giving us some riding instruction in the arena. With this new focus, I had lost track of my feelings about Dove. Eventually, the other horses and riders returned down the narrow path. My heart sank again. I remember not being surprised when my group was told that Dove had been a "problem" on the trail. I remember thinking to myself, "I could have told you that!" I sat and fumed over how little anyone really seemed to care about this poor guy or about his condition.

On Thursday, the final full day of the clinic, I was relieved to find that no one had been assigned to ride Dove. "Yeah," I thought to myself, "maybe somebody's finally got it." The air was light as we all knew we were almost through. We had spent a lot of time in the saddle over the week, learned a lot about instructing and made some good buddies in the process. After lunch, it was announced that our final afternoon session would concentrate on cantering examples. Returning to the arena, I was dismayed to find Dove, now my emotional focus of the week, included yet again in the afternoon session. As the horses entered the arena for the afternoon session, all I could do was sit and watch. Only a few horse and rider combinations were going to be chosen to provide a cantering example for the rest of the group that afternoon; Dove and his rider were one of them. At his turn, he was brought forward out of the line of other horses. After only a few seconds of walking along the rail, the clinic leader requested that Dove's rider should ask him to proceed into a trot. Then, after the rider had been given careful instruction on where to pick up the correct lead for the canter, Dove was about to be asked to comply. He came around the corner and the rider cued for the canter but, instead of complying with his rider's demands, he became flustered and stayed in a trot; now trotting as fast as he could. The leader asked the rider to stop and to try the maneuver again but the same pattern emerged and once again, Dove refused to pick up the canter. He would only trot. They asked her to try again.

As I sat there watching, I could clearly see and *feel* what the challenge was. The more it went on, the more I could feel it. It was as if my own body was in pain and screaming inside, "But it hurts."

As I listened again to the instructions being called out to the rider, I became conscious of the fact that the instructor thought Dove needed to be corrected. I watched him suffer for what seemed to be an endless amount of time; I could see he was in pain as plain as day and I knew in my heart of hearts that he was not trying to be disrespectful, *he was hurting*. It was on that particular day in June, at that very moment, that my passion showed itself to me with complete clarity.

Dove was pulled to a stop and without hesitation, the instructor called out, "Go get a crop." Seething, I realized that her answer to the situation was to whip him into compliance, under any circumstance. I was overwhelmed. With secret tears flowing under my sunglasses, I couldn't look at him, but only down at the ground. I wanted to scream: *"before you take a crop to the poor animal, why don't you find out what's really going on!"* After a few seconds, I looked up and had no choice but to watch this thoughtless act of cruelty. I could see the look of shock and confusion that Dove had in his eyes. His *real* problem was so clear to me, yet the other nine people in the arena didn't seem to even notice. As Dove (bless his heart), stoic in spite of his pain, submitted to his rider, it seemed to me that I could feel every painful stride with him. My mood was changed for the rest of the day. It was all I could think about and I was so mad at the disservice to the poor animal. I realized later that my commitment to horses grew stronger in that moment and changed me forever.

After a long sleepless night of thinking things over and feeling such an aversion to what I'd seen, Friday arrived. The final session was to be a morning of wrapping things up and distributing certifications. We all waited for our turn to have a private consultation with the two group leaders: I chose to be the last to go. I contemplated whether I should try to explain my true feelings and share my observations over the week. In the end, I chose to speak up for Dove. This was my chance. My summary of the week to them went like this;

- Monday, the horse exhibited back pain, yet was ridden anyway.
- On Tuesday, he did get a break, for *one* day. I told them I suspected his back pain was due to a vertebra or rib being out of alignment, as I had experienced this on my own horse, or maybe an ill-fitting saddle.
- Wednesday he was labeled "a problem" on the trail but I knew that the down hill maneuvering had simply aggravated his back pain whether it was a rib or saddle fit.
- Thursday's cantering challenge was so clear to me. He was not trying to disobey the rider, nor was it that the rider was not cueing him correctly for the canter, it was that he was hurting. His inability or refusal to pick up the canter was purely because he was in pain.

I was saddened that my observations about Dove seemed to fall on deaf ears. It felt to me as if the two leaders could not admit to maybe missing something. As I drove away that Friday afternoon, I realized that in spite of my attempts to inform the "higher ups" about an obvious oversight of Dove's condition, I was not heard or even understood. It was overwhelming knowing that they missed the mark on Dove's problem. If only folks would take the time to consider a horse's condition, maybe a horse's life or relationship with a rider could be made better. Although I did feel a sense of accomplishment in having completed the course and in being certified as an instructor, it was overshadowed by my sadness for Dove. What would his life be like from there forward? It was apparent to me that the biggest challenge for Dove, and for so many other horses, was his inability to describe or communicate his pain to a population of humans who simply didn't know, didn't understand, or didn't care.

Fast forward to today. I am a continuing student and have studied many things on behalf of the horse that might be misunderstood when it comes to a horse's behavior. Even my own horse, Grace, has been an eye-opening example of understanding simple miscalculations. My findings over time included ribs, vertebra and pelvic joints out of alignment, inappropriate shoeing, poor-fitting saddles, and severe tension and stress in muscles. I also found bits that did not fit and were inappropriate for Grace's age and level of training, and lastly, dental work that left her jaw locked at the temporomandibular joint, also known as the TMJ. As a consequence to some of these conditions, she couldn't hold a canter well, wouldn't pick up leads, twisted her rear feet when walking, hollowed out in the back during the canter, had muscle atrophy where the saddle was bearing down, was mouthy, and was unable to collect correctly due to the jaw being unable to move backwards. Although Grace was asked to perform under many such conditions, she did her job in spite of it all.

I now feel strongly that it's our responsibility to educate ourselves to be able to meet the requirements of our own horses. The natural cooperative spirit of a horse will give us its best when its needs are met. In our modern approach, we

have grossly underestimated the intuitiveness and intelligence of our horses. We, as owners, must do our own research on these basic topics of comfort for our horse's sake.

My ambition is to keep learning so that I can be a strong advocate for the horse. I am not trying to say that all people are irresponsible or uncaring. There are many good horsemen and horsewomen out there with lots of experience in these areas. My goal is to help anyone who is having trouble, perhaps through a lack of understanding, to help bridge the gap that might possibly exist in communication between them and their horse. I think these ideas defined in one book just might help expose the common elements of confusion that can lead to a horse being labeled a "problem" through no fault of its own. What we perceive to be "bad behavior" is very often the result of poor handling, improper equipment or any number of physiological conditions that our horses are unable to describe to us.

According to the American Horse Council, the horse industry is a 102 billion dollar industry annually. Although the racing industry is typically known for the largest segment of contribution, close to 4 million horses are now involved in recreational riding pursuits and close to 3 million of those owners are competing or showing annually. In all, it is estimated that over 7 million people work in or around the horse industry. I feel it is *our duty and responsibility* to invest the time and energy into learning about proper care and the concerns of our horses.

In this book, I provide basic but essential information, using an eight-item checklist that can be used any time you are having an off day or when things just seem to be amiss. No matter how experienced we are, we always need to check and re-check each of these components before blaming the horse. I believe that if most riders would adopt this attitude toward preparing for or reviewing a ride, our horses would be so much better for it. Unfortunately, in the world of riding, it's my experience that even seasoned horse owners or trainers can fail to assess the *real* issues behind why they are experiencing a "bumpy ride" with their horses. All too often, the horse is blamed and suffers the consequences. Our challenge is to make a concerted effort to understand some of the pain these stoic animals may be enduring on our behalf before blaming them for their behavior.

We can find very in-depth information on the multiple topics outlined here for our own study. I encourage you to do your own research and continue to study the subjects discussed in this book and to expand your knowledge. Sadly, I have witnessed plenty of people who choose to look at their horse as nothing more than an object there to serve them. This book is *not* for them.

This book is for the owner who believes somewhere in their soul that their partner, the horse, deserves the best thought and care possible.

I have read several how-to books that provide wonderful information on the broad care of horses, but felt there was a lack of reading material that focused specifically on ways a horse might be experiencing pain; pain that prohibits them from providing a satisfying ride without suffering.

I want to address the most common areas of misunderstanding in ride preparation and in good general care, and present them in one book. I consider all of the physiology-based components described in this book to be instrumental in understanding equine behavior. Signs of poor behavior might actually be signs of more than one source of pain or irritation, subtle or not so subtle. Any of the areas of concern discussed in the following chapters, either singularly or combined, can be the *real* source of behavioral issues, more times than we think. It's advisable to check them all or at least consider them, to eliminate doubt.

When our horses are not cooperating, instead of presuming it is bad behavior, consider that it might be due to discomfort or pain they are experiencing.

As we all know, there are so many different ideas about ways to do things with our horses, some good and some bad. I certainly don't have all the answers to every equine behavior challenge, but my hope is that horse owners will start to look at things "outside the box." These misunderstandings can make or break their relationship with their horse. I have seen folks more interested in owning fancy trucks, trailers, tack or other such items of prestige, including their horses, rather than investing time in getting to know and understand the living creature that so willingly carries them. In addition, many hours and dollars are sometimes spent on riding instruction or training in an effort to improve performance without the slightest thought given to things outside the horse's control. By taking the time to ensure that your horse is comfortable and *able* to do what is being asked of him or her effectively, you will be doing your horse a great service. The more you know and understand your own horse, the more confident you can be that you are able to provide the best care needed. Increasing your own knowledge also makes it possible to find reputable and proven experts in your particular area when you do need help.

Choosing to follow a path of learning is a true demonstration of your desire to be the best horseman, owner, rider, or trainer you can possibly be. In choosing to at least examine the ideas in this book, you are showing your enthusiasm for learning how to be the best partner you can be with the horse. With dignity and love, I hope that these ideas open up a door to a wonderful new relationship between you and your horse. This type of a relationship is one that only a human who truly cares about his or her horse can truly have.

CHAPTER 1

Understanding Your Horse's Legs and Good Basic Shoeing

Horses were created by the best designer in the world, and that design, for the most part, is flawless. It is man who over time has interfered and changed, or at least tried to redesign, the modern horse. Large bodies on small, refined legs and feet represent one example of a man-made change. Under the conditions in which we expect our horses to perform, and in doing the many maneuvers we expect of them, we've moved away from nature's intended use of a horse's feet and legs. We don't seem to give this very much consideration until our horse comes up lame.

Steel shoes and concrete floors have removed the horse from its natural connection with the earth.

Without going into a complete anatomical explanation, it can be said that the legs are a complex composite of finely integrated parts that from the beginning of time have served the horse well. The hoof is a finely tuned instrument that can withstand rock, sand, movement at 25 mph and tolerate miles and miles of traveling every day for many years; it is also pliable, supple and water resistant, yet it's light enough to lift. Many supplements are sold to "strengthen" horse's hooves. Supplements *can* help, but actually, it is movement that builds the hoof wall.

Hoof and Leg Function

As humans, we all move differently; we have different shaped legs, different ways of walking, and different gaits. We know that certain biomechanical issues such as flat footedness, high arches, hammer toes, etc. can lead to localized or referred pain in the course of everyday movements and manifest into overuse injuries in human athletes. However, with that said, a flatfooted athlete can still become an Olympic champion. All of the above issues are totally treatable and can be managed to allow pain free movement. This exact same approach can be applied to our horses in terms of overcoming faults in order to achieve optimum hoof and leg function. Of course, issues can only be managed once they are recognized. That's why it's important that we understand good conformation and any problems our horses may have in relation to hoof and leg function due to conformation faults. Taking steps to correct biomechanical issues causing pain or difficulty with certain movements is critical to soundness and longevity.

Legs are made up of bones, joints, muscles, tendons and ligaments, nervous, vascular and lymphatic systems. Size or breed do not change the basic structure, but other hereditary features can affect the way a horse's legs and feet function, as can their overall physical and mental state. Our own involvement as human partners aboard can also have an influence on the horse, to be addressed later. The point I'm making is that a horse doesn't necessarily need to possess "perfect" conformation to be the perfect horse for you. Human athletes come in all shapes and sizes, and it's the same with equine athletes. Making the most of what we have is the key to enjoying freedom of movement in our everyday activities, whether that's preparing for an afternoon on the trail or preparing for the Olympics. Our horses can't tell us what they are feeling so we must learn to pay attention to the small signs and symptoms that can lead to much bigger problems if we fail to recognize them.

I often wonder why it is that some people can completely overlook poor hoof condition in their horses, but if they found a blemish on the coat or skin, they would be on the search for an immediate remedy. By paying close attention to the hooves, we can learn a great deal about the movement of our horses. The hoof not only shows signs of how a horse moves, it actually records those moves like a map. It's amazing to me that a horse can recover from some of the extreme lameness and trauma they experience. The message I want to convey in this chapter is that although many things can contribute to lameness, it's something that *can often be prevented.* Our responsibility as caring horse owners is to educate ourselves and to understand conditions that might lead to lameness. The more we *know* our horses, the better we can care for them.

> **BEFORE THE CROP COMES OUT…KEY POINT TO CONSIDER NUMBER 1**
>
> **SOUND HOOVES AND LEGS HELP TO CREATE A FULLY FUNCTIONAL HORSE.**

Is Your Horse a Sound, Fully Functioning Horse?

Not all lameness is immediately obvious. If your horse is unable to put a hoof to the ground or if contact with the ground is causing a visible, painful reaction, making any forward movement virtually impossible, then your horse is *clearly* lame. However, the absence of *obvious* lameness doesn't necessarily mean your horse is sound. To be a sound and fully functional horse, he or she needs an even rhythm in every gait along with balance and suppleness; they need to be fully focused, self confident, vibrant, coordinated, willing to go forward and must be fully conditioned to their level of training.

Among the things that can contribute to lameness are:

Infection – This can result from bad husbandry, wounds or diseases.

Trauma – Either physical trauma from an incident or mental trauma from fear; fear from an event, fear from pain, fear from reprimand.

Degeneration – Declining over time and with age.

Metabolic disorders – Includes conditions such as equine Cushing's disorder, Laminitis or Azoturia (tying up).

Allergies – These can cause inflammation as the body reacts to reject something.

Hereditary – Genetic conformation faults passed on from parents.

Developmental disorders – May include dietary imbalances, poor conditioning, stress or early accidents.

I believe that stress can cause tension, and that our horses today carry too much undiscovered stress. Tension can have a negative impact on the way a horse moves and therefore can contribute to potential lameness. The need for bodywork to relieve tension in the horse is discussed further in chapter two.

Not all of the above factors can be avoided or prevented but they can all be *managed* and in most cases carefully controlled to give a horse the best chance of enjoying a fully functional life. Of course, this means they must first be recognized.

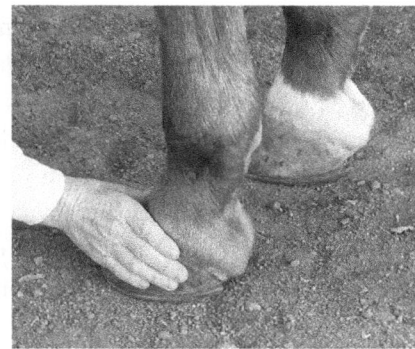

Figure 1.1 Feel each hoof for even or similar temperatures. If one feels different than the others, this might be a potential sign of trouble.

Checking for Lameness

In looking for lameness, begin by checking the temperature of each hoof with your hand (Fig. 1.1). A hot or cold hoof might indicate a problem. Other symptoms to look for are heat or cold in other areas on the body (Fig. 1.2), numbness and swelling, lack of range of motion, muscle tension, or deformation. Anything that strikes you as abnormal is going to help you find answers to questions of soundness. This means *knowing* your horse and recognizing not only physical changes but also changes in mood or attitude.

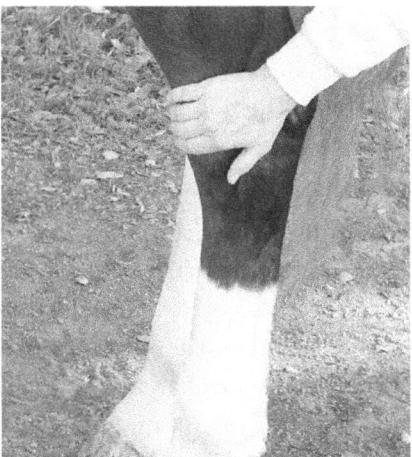

Figure 1.2 Check other parts of the body for heat, swelling, knots or anything that seems abnormal.

Look with your eyes.
Listen with your ears and your heart.
Feel with your hands and your gut instinct.
Analyze with your head, your intellect, and your intuition.

The more in tune you become with your horse, the more you will develop your ability to trust your gut feeling and sense when something isn't right.

Other Contributing Factors to Lameness

- **Standing surface**

  The surface that your horse stands on daily, in the stall or elsewhere, makes a big difference to your horse. Some folks have horses stand on concrete for long periods of time, yet if standing there themselves, would find themselves shifting uncomfortably from foot to foot until they eventually felt the need to sit down. Why is it that we don't seem to have the same consideration for our horses? Stall mats, for example, are fine for outdoor paddocks in winter as long as there is comfortable ground to stand or lie down on elsewhere. Typically, mats are not recommended in the summer heat as they radiate that heat up and through the hooves. It's my experience that black stall mats in the dead of summer become so hot to the touch, that for the horse, it must feel similar to us walking barefoot on a hot asphalt road.

- **Circulation**

  Nutrients are delivered via water yet water does not travel uphill. Horses that stand still for hours in a stall need to get out daily, and need the help of a flexible ground surface to aid circulation and keep fluid moving back up the leg and around the body. Many horses are expected to stand motionless in a stall for long periods and then immediately go to work as soon as someone gets them out, without any time for gradual circulation increase. Horses need to take it slow and an appropriate warm up period is essential at the beginning of any ride – further details can be found in chapter 7.

- **Riding surface**

  Pasture horses are already adapted to handling rolling terrain, but for a stalled horse that doesn't get much exercise, coming out on uneven ground can be an accident waiting to happen. It is important to allow a horse time to adjust to footing or terrain (familiar or unfamiliar) and let them figure out how best to maneuver in it. Riding on asphalt roads also requires careful conditioning to prepare the tendons and ligaments. It's important to understand that a steel shoe on slippery asphalt does not grip. When a horse feels unable to grasp the surface they're walking on, they will naturally tend to tense their muscles just as you or I would if we found ourselves slipping on an icy surface.

Horses need time to adjust to variations in arena or road footing. If your horse is used to only one or two types of riding surface, changing to another can represent an entirely different need to adjust physically. New footing represents new muscle use and new confidence, especially if there are significant changes in depth or in surface materials.

- **Our need to exert our own authority over our horse**

  In times past, the ancient Greeks paid as much attention to the development of their horse as they did to their own physical and mental development. We, only in our recent past, have finally begun to realize that horses are no longer our servants but willing partners. Maybe some of their moods or off days should be taken into consideration. Still, today many people don't seem to understand that their horse's body is an extension of their own. In her book, *Understanding the Horse's Legs*, Sara Wyche mentions cases of rough controlling handlers with back pain or arthritic hands whose horse suffers similar back pain or forehand lameness due to the link between the two. In addition, a rider who is stiff and inflexible himself can somehow find it hard to believe that their horse just might be experiencing the same thing.

Before reprimanding your horse for unwillingness to move forwards, consider whether they may actually be **unsure** *or* **unable,** *not unwilling.*

Basic Shoeing

We've taught our horses that they need to be shod, and over time they've become dependent on shoes. They watch our mannerisms and our expectations because they are interested in pleasing us. They adapt to wearing shoes because we want them to, even though it's far removed from what nature intended. Horses adjust and learn how to grip in shoes but if you've ever tried walking in someone else's boots and have experienced the feel of unfamiliar heel angles or wear, you'll have some understanding of how new or incorrect shoes might feel to a horse. Just as your new riding boots may need a breaking-in period before they feel totally comfortable, a horse also needs time to adjust to the feel of new shoes each time they are shod. This is especially important if you make any changes in shoe style, or major adjustments in your normal shoeing cycle.

Most horse owners are unaware of the importance of having a critical eye for shoeing. A farrier is thought of as a mechanic, but he or she should really be considered more like a surgeon. Everything a farrier does will affect the balance of the bones inside the hoof, and all the way up the leg. If it's not done correctly, the horse suffers. Without the correct balance in the hoof, the internal bones can be traumatized and the tendons and ligaments can be put under unnecessary strain. Some owners do put some time and effort into looking at shoeing angles from a side view by looking for correct

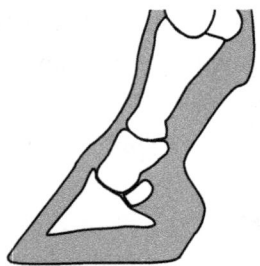

Figure 1.3 Correct bone alignment from the side.

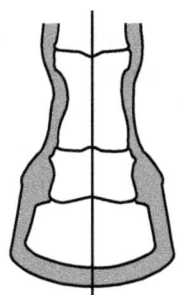

Figure 1.4 Correct bone alignment from the front.

alignment of the bones (Fig. 1.3), but we don't often pay much attention to balance issues that can only be diagnosed from a straight on, front view. If you look at wild horses, they often have heels that are far from picture perfect yet they are not lame. A closer look at the same horses from a front view reveals that they are always centered and in balance over the center of each hoof (Fig. 1.4). Unfortunately, the same can't be said for our domestically shod horses. This is due to some less than desirable shoeing procedures being done today. Horses develop a "hand" bias as humans do. Horses, like people, become right-handed or left-handed. Our one-sidedness as riders and uneven riding tendencies are picked up by the sensitive horse, and our strengths and weaknesses in the saddle inevitably contribute to the development of stronger or weaker sides in the horse. This does not benefit the balance of the hoof nor does it benefit the back, shoulder, stifle, hock, etc. It takes much more energy to stand on an uneven surface than a level one and as the horse moves, energy is translated up the leg to the bones and joints, often putting more pressure on one side of the horse. Again, shoeing is of utmost importance in this area. If the horse's energy or motion is out of alignment or balance for any reason, it can lead to unwanted issues (Fig. 1.5 and Fig 1.6).

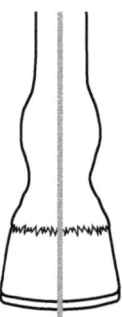

Figure 1.5 Even lateral balance of the hoof from the front. The leg is centered over the hoof.

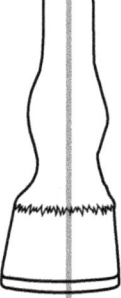

Figure 1.6 Uneven lateral balance of the hoof from the front. The leg is NOT centered over the hoof.

Basic Shoeing Check

To do a basic check for balanced shoeing, square your horse up on level ground and position yourself to view them from the front.

- Imagine the front of your horse as a picture frame with the chest, the inside edge of the front legs, and the ground creating the frame (Fig. 1.7).
- Look for symmetry; are the knees even in height? A lot of horses have one leg longer or shorter than the other (Fig. 1.8) and it's not uncommon to find horses have completely different sized feet (Fig. 1.9).

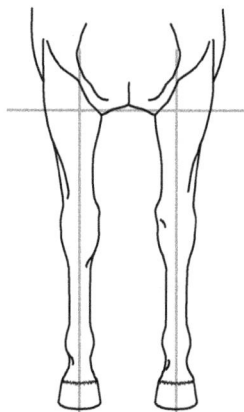

Figure 1.7 Example of how to view the front legs as a picture frame.

Draw an imaginary line from the knee, through the canon bone, through the fetlock, down the pastern and then through the hoof to the ground. You should find there is an equal amount of hoof on each side of that line in all four hooves (Fig. 1.10).

- View the heel angles of the front feet by looking at them from about a 45-degree angle from behind the heels; are the heels even in height (Fig. 1.11). Many horses have a lower or higher heel (Fig. 1.12) and I have learned and discovered on my own horse that this can cause an over-development of the shoulder muscles on the side of the body with the lower heel. It may also be that the one-sidedness of the rider is another contributing factor to uneven muscle development.

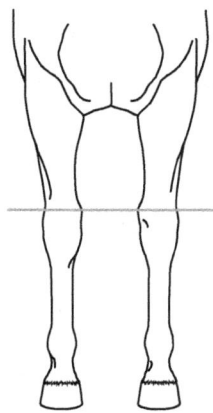

Figure 1.8 Check for level knees on a level surface.

- Take a look at the coronet bands. Make sure they are all completely level and in line with the ground, not tilting one way or another. Again, this must be done on level ground to be accurate (Fig. 1.13).

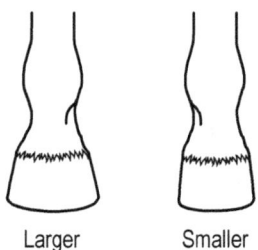

Larger   Smaller

Figure 1.9 Check for even sized feet.

UNDERSTANDING YOUR HORSE'S LEGS AND GOOD BASIC SHOEING

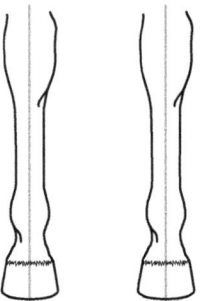

Figure 1.10 When a line is drawn from the knee through the front of the cannon bone and down through the hoof, there should be equal amounts of hoof on either side of the line.

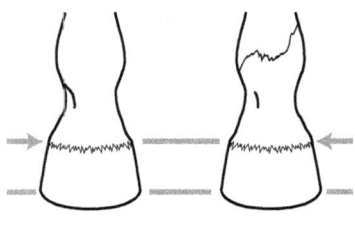

Figure 1.13 Check for level coronet bands.

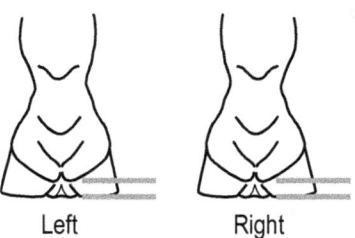

Figure 1.11 View heels from the rear at a 45 degree angle. Are the heel heights matching between both front feet and both rear feet?

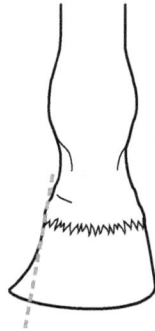

Figure 1.14 Check for flares or other deformities.

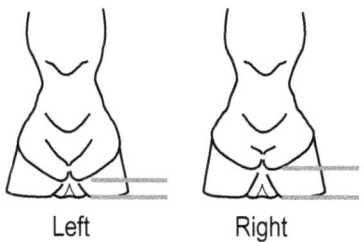

Figure 1.12 Check for differences in heel height.

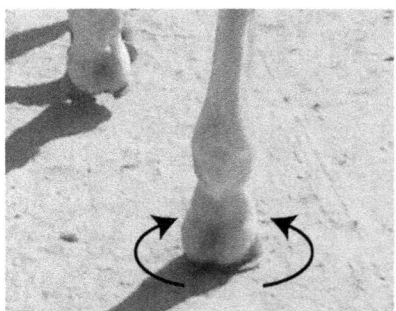

Figure 1.15 Look for any twisting movement in the hoof while walking the horse in a straight line.

- Look for flares; does the hoof shape appear to flare out towards the bottom on one side or the other? This is typically due to an over-long medial (inside) or lateral (outside) hoof wall (Fig. 1.14).
- Have someone walk the horse so you can view his or her movement coming toward you and going away from you. Is there a twisting movement in any of the hooves? This can be another indicator of an uneven medial or lateral side (Fig. 1.15).

- Observe the hoof position as it hits the ground; does the hoof land flat or does one side connect with the ground before the other? Each hoof should land completely flat.
- Pick up the hoof to measure for symmetry. Begin by measuring from the center of the frog to the front of the hoof and then center of the frog to the back of the hoof. These distances should be equal. You should also measure from the center of the frog to the right and to

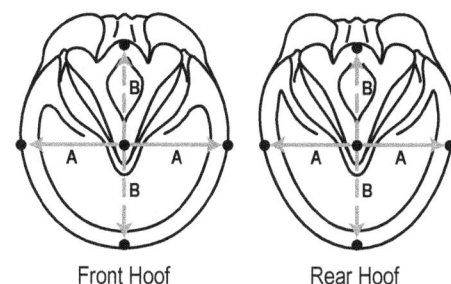

Figure 1.16 Balanced distances from the center of the frog. Hoof should be viewed barefoot, without horseshoes, if possible. Rear feet should measure slightly narrower than the front feet. This is normal.

the left (side to side). The distances should be equal except in the rear hooves. The hind hooves are generally narrower in shape and that is natural (Fig. 1.16). In the front hooves, all four measurements should be close, creating a symmetrical shape. Ideally, the measurements should be done barefoot as perimeter shoes can distort the measurement if they hang over the side of a hoof at all. A balanced hoof is the best condition for a normal hoof and leg.

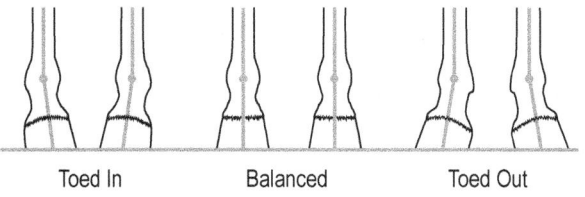

Figure 1.17 Common conformation flaws in the horse are feet that are toed in or toed out.

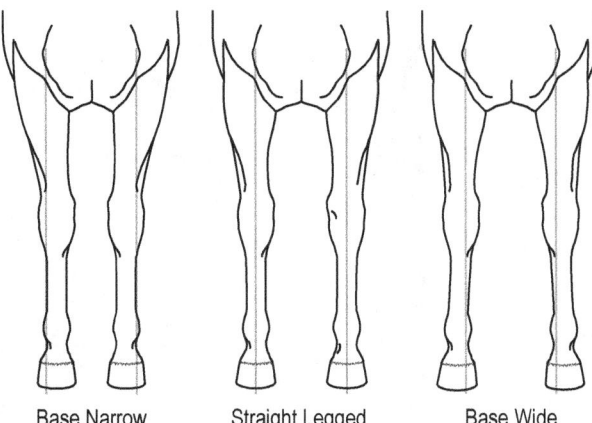

Figure 1.18 Additional conformation flaws include the horse standing base narrow or base wide.

Of course not all horses have perfect conformation to begin with. Where there are already existing conformation flaws, such as being toed in or toed out (Fig. 1.17), base narrow or base wide (Fig. 1.18), there's a need to do a bit of adjusting to create the ideal balance in each hoof. This is where a good farrier is worth his or her weight in gold. The more you educate yourself and understand *your* horse and its feet, the more able you are to have a well-informed discussion with your farrier and to determine your horse's needs.

Owner Responsibilities

Farriers nowadays typically don't have time to assess muscle development. Many good farriers can tell a lot by the hoof itself, but it's up to us as owners and riders to notice any changes and describe them to our farriers. This means we need to pay close attention to the art of shoeing and the movement and stride of our horses in order to be able to translate our findings to the farrier. It can be helpful to watch your horse's movements on a lunge line without tack. Does he or she appear to be laboring in a particular a gait? Is there an unevenness of rhythm? Does one or more of the legs fail to come up underneath as far as the other? Do the front legs seem fluid, even and elongated? Understanding rhythm and developing an eye for balance and stride does take a bit of time. I suggest watching videos that demonstrate sound gait movement to compare what you see with your own horse's strides. Each horse and breed is different, so take time to learn all you can by watching as many other horses as possible.

There are so many choices of shoes now in use that we can't go into an in-depth description of each in this one short chapter. Each has its own characteristic and vibration. The amount of vibration experienced by the horse in each case is difficult to determine but it undoubtedly has an effect. The hoof is an organ; it's a gauge of health. It could be something as small as a tiny vibration in the hoof that might have a major effect on the entire horse. To ensure our horses remain fully functional, we must begin to pay more attention to their hoof care on a daily basis, not just when things go wrong.

Grace's Story

When my horse, Grace, was brought into training, we took lower leg and hoof x-rays. These revealed that her bone axis was broken back (Fig. 1.19), meaning that the long and short pastern bones and coffin bone were not in alignment as they should be. The only way to correct this was to put her in a high heel shoe called a degree shoe (Fig. 1.20). The vet recommended that she wear a three-degree shoe to correct the amount of misalignment. The degree shoe is supposed to be a temporary fix for most horses until the heels can grow again, creating the correct alignment. It's important to note here that some breeds don't grow heel well or at all, thus emphasizing the need to engage a good farrier in the first place.

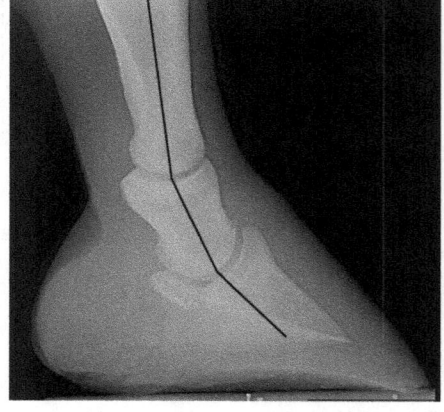

Figure 1.19 Grace before – note broken angles.

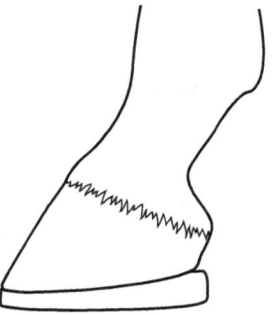

Figure 1.20 Degree shoe.

Grace's degree correction made perfect sense to me. However, because the farrier couldn't locate a three-degree shoe, Grace was initially put in a two-degree shoe with one degree of padding. It was then suggested that we could change that to a one-degree shoe with two degrees of padding for more softness and comfort. Unfortunately, at that time I didn't understand the use of pads. We did new x-rays six months later, hoping she had grown some heel, but nothing had changed. We concluded then that due to the lack of new heel growth, Grace would have to wear degree shoes for the rest of her life.

I felt the need to understand and study hoof balance for myself and learned that a horse will *not* grow heel while wearing pads. Wedge pads actually crush the heels underneath so they are unable to grow. Eventually Grace's farrier found a three-degree aluminum shoe to use. This was optimal for the farrier, as it would save him time and labor not having to cut and assemble pads at each shoeing. It was optimal for Grace, too. After she wore these shoes for well over a year, it began to look to my new farrier that she actually *had* grown heel. The farrier suggested we do new x-rays and low and behold, she was back to a normal alignment (Fig. 1.21). We then began dropping her out of the degree shoes one degree at a time. This slow dropping process is *very* important as tendons need time to stretch out to their new length. I also discovered that Grace had one heel shorter than the other. My farrier and I then chose to move down in degrees with different height shoes i.e. a two degree on one front foot and a one degree on the other to balance the horse. Her lower heeled shoulder was very pronounced which is actually common. Since dropping her into regular shoes, the shoulder has changed dramatically. We still believe that her front left leg is a bit longer than her right leg causing her heel on the left to grow slightly different from the heel on the right due to hitting the ground first and hardest. Besides the new heel growth, Grace also had a twisting action in her rear hooves when she walked in a straight line. During my study of balanced shoeing, I learned that her twisting was probably because of a long lateral (outside edge) side

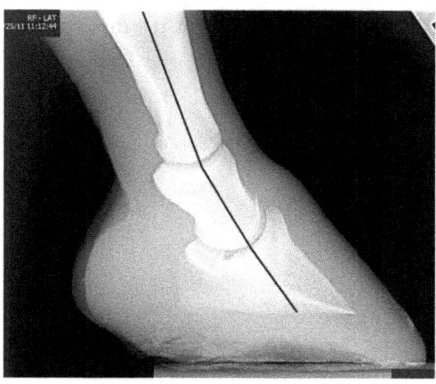

Figure 1.21 Grace after – notice the improved angles and the additional heel growth.

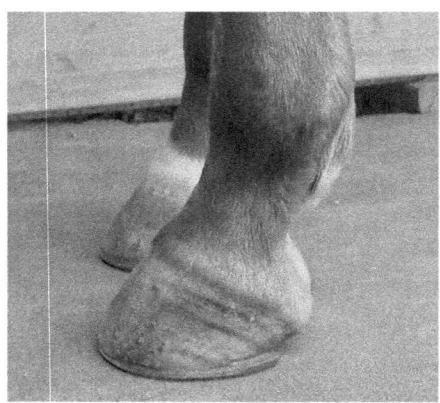

Figure 1.22 Grace today – in regular flat shoes.

grabbing the ground first. When this was confirmed by my new farrier, and corrected with a balanced trim, the twist no longer existed. Grace, after several resets, is now wearing regular flat shoes on both front feet (Fig. 1.22), moving better than she ever has and the left shoulder is slowly shrinking, beginning to match the right shoulder more.

I wanted to expand my thinking about any contributing factors that affect movement so I pursued some training in tension release work (see chapter two). Along with needing shoeing changes, I discovered that Grace had severe tension in the poll area, the neck area, the shoulders and the hind leg area. The tension release training was eye opening for me and it all began to make sense, in terms of putting the picture together. I became aware that Grace could not reach out well with her front legs and appeared to be stabbing the ground each time she took a step. After lowering her out of degree shoes, and doing many sessions of tension release work, she is able to stride well out in front of herself and canter much longer than she ever could. I believe that this is due to the shoeing changes and from freeing up those muscles, tendons and ligaments allowing them to move more freely.

Grace's story suggests that we shouldn't just leave a check for the farrier, and then simply trust the results. We need to be educated and involved in shoeing decisions and be on the team of people responsible for our horse. The more you increase your own understanding of *your* horse's hooves, legs and movement, the more likely it is that you will help make the correct shoeing decisions for your horse the first time. The bottom line is that a farrier can shoe your horse but until you educate yourself, it's difficult for you to know if the farrier has done a good job or if it's the *best* that can be done for your horse's sake.

CHAPTER 2

Why Chiropractic and Massage

When I first purchased my horse, everything was going well. One day though, I noticed that she was unwilling to pick up the right lead to a lope. I started to feel that it was something I was doing wrong; I wondered if I might be throwing her off balance in some way. The more it became an issue, the less confident I felt. What was I doing wrong? The turning point came one day when her difficulty with picking up the lead escalated into a bucking episode that took me completely by surprise. This behavior wasn't something I had experienced with her before. I sought out a local trainer that I admired who had an intuitive understanding of horses. She told me a story about a horse with a bad back that really helped shape my understanding of the need for chiropractic care and massage therapy. The horse would ride along fine for the most part, but when a trainer asked him to collect, he would go crazy. Several trainers had tried to work through his 'behavioral issues' but would end up giving up on him, saying he was "too much of a problem." Some recommended that he be retired. He was finally brought to my trainer's facility. She had an equine chiropractor come to check him out. The chiropractor figured out that the horse had a back vertebra out of alignment, which was pinching a nerve and sending a shooting pain down his rear legs every time he tried to tuck his head to collect. After being adjusted by the chiropractor, over time the issue was resolved and he ended up becoming a good riding horse.

What is Equine Chiropractic?

I know that some people are skeptical of chiropractic care for horses. For some there is good reason. Most likely they've had a bad experience, or have heard stories of being taken advantage of. Although there are the "experts" who give the practice a bad name, we as humans find benefit all the time from chiropractic care. If we were to look at a horse's anatomy standing upright on its hind legs, we'd find that there's not much difference between humans and horses. The philosophy behind chiropractic therapy is that the body has an innate ability to heal itself. The whole body, whether equine or human, is controlled by the nervous system. The core belief in chiropractic treatment is that subluxation (a joint that has moved out of its normal position) can lead to the surrounding nerves becoming pinched. This will interfere with the body's ability to function as intended. Although the joint has moved, unlike a dislocation, it hasn't moved enough to prevent it from functioning totally. A subluxation often results in a limited range of movement and a level of discomfort that might be described by a human sufferer as anything from plain "back pain" to a "pinched nerve." There are a lot of areas on a horse's body where subluxation can occur, but the most common is the spine. This slight misalignment of the bones can be caused by a variety of factors, but the added unnatural weight of a saddle and rider on a horse's back can undoubtedly be a potential contributing factor. This highlights the importance of having a correctly fitted saddle, a consideration discussed further in chapter 3. Of course, subluxation in any of your horse's joints can cause the same level of discomfort we as humans might experience, but the only way the horse can communicate their difficulty is through their behavior.

Behavioral Issues Connected to Subluxation
- Lameness.
- A noticeable change in gait.
- Unwilling to perform a certain action, such as picking up a particular lead at the canter or lope.
- Irritability.
- Short striding action.

> **BEFORE THE CROP COMES OUT...KEY POINT TO CONSIDER**
> **NUMBER 2**
>
> **RESISTANCE OR DIFFICULTY IN MOVEMENT COULD BE THE RESULT OF HIDDEN TENSION OR PAIN.**

Finding Hidden Pain

If you are experiencing behavioral issues with your horse, it is essential that you take steps to locate any hidden sites of pain so that subluxation and associated challenges can either be eliminated from your list of potential causes or identified and treated appropriately to provide relief. This is a three step process that begins with a chiropractic back check.

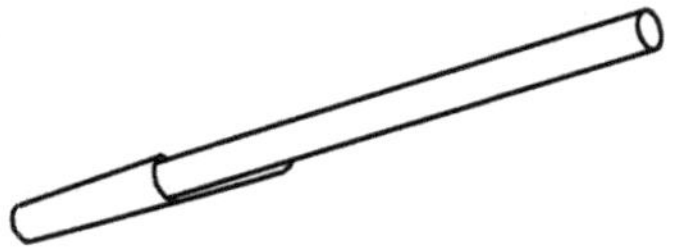

Figure 2.1 A basic pen with cap can be used for a simple back check.

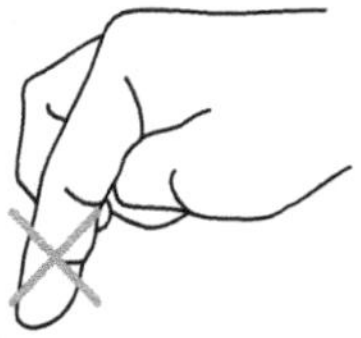

Figure 2.2 Do not use your fingertips as the results will not be the same.

Step One:
Simple Chiropractic Back Check

To do a basic check on your horse's back, all you need is a firm, round-ended object such as a pen with a cap. Fingertips or finger-nails are not suitable (Fig. 2.1 and Fig. 2.2)

- Begin by identifying the gap of around one hand's width between the top of your horse's withers and the top of their shoulder blade or scapula. The center of that area is then the starting point for your back check. (Fig. 2.3)
- Using the pen with a cap, or similar object, find your starting point, again about an inch and a half away from the spine. Begin by making short strokes of three to four inches along the back, applying the same pressure you would use to write with. (Fig. 2.4)
- Stay consistent as you move along the back to stay about an inch and a half away from the spine. This checking procedure goes all the way up and over the pelvic area almost to the tail. (Fig. 2.5) If you find your horse responds by dipping his or her back, you might have located a potential problem area. (Fig. 2.6)
- If the reaction area is four to six inches in length, this most likely indicates a muscle related or soreness issue. A dip response generated over a smaller area of approximately one to two inches indicates there may be a potential bone adjustment needed.
- This procedure or check should be done on both sides of the spine.

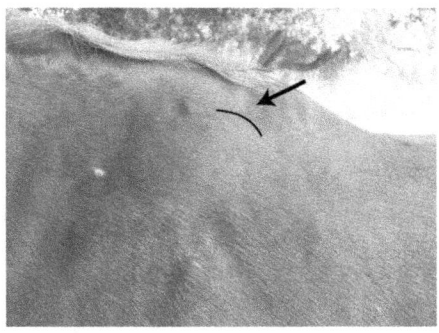

Figure 2.3 Starting point is halfway between the top of the withers and the top of the scapula. Be sure that the top of your horse's scapula is approximately one human hand width from the wither. A smaller measurement might indicate a raised scapula needing to address as a chiropractic issue of its own.

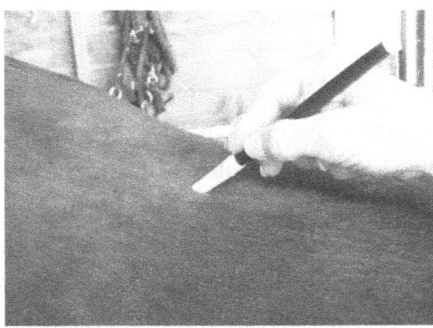

Figure 2.4 Begin making short strokes about 3 to 4 inches in length. Use the pressure you would use in writing on paper.

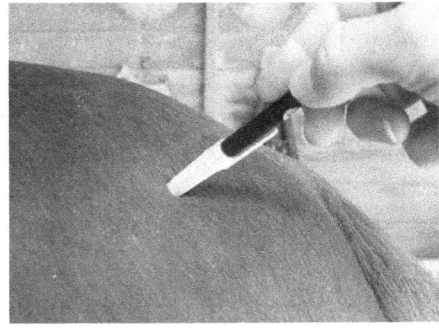

Figure 2.5 Check the back approximately 1 and ½ inch off the spine all the way back to the base of the tail.

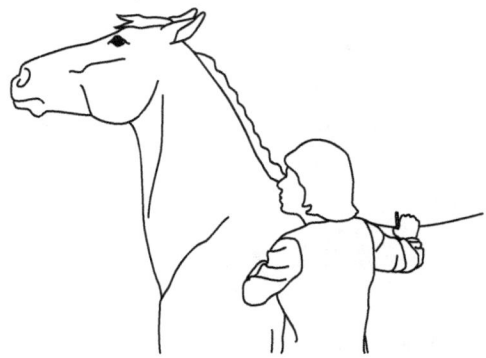

Figure 2.6 A response showing a potential problem.

Any subluxations you notice or concerns you have can then be thoroughly checked out and corrected by a reputable chiropractor. It is important to find a chiropractor that both you and your horse feel comfortable with. Effective chiropractic therapy goes beyond just acquiring a certified qualification; it takes a practitioner with real-life experience and an *intuitive* understanding of each horse they treat as an individual, to generate lasting, positive results. I feel that it is important to locate a professional who has advanced training in chiropractic and a number of years of experience doing numerous adjustments.

Step Two:

Checking for Muscle Tension

Subluxation can also cause pain in the muscles surrounding the affected bones, as they must work harder to support the movement of the joint. Pain then leads to tension, often resulting in referred pain. Referred pain is pain perceived at a location other than the site of the painful stimulus. An example of referred pain in humans would be the pain commonly felt in the left arm in the case of a heart attack. Tension can develop elsewhere in the body as a result of other muscle groups being recruited to compensate for the consequent changes or limitations in movement. Of course, tension in a horse's muscles can also simply be the result of an intense workout, just as in our own muscles, so it's important to consider whether the pressures placed on your horse's body during your last training session or ride may be having a residual effect on your current session. A human athlete needs recovery time after a period of intense training and your horse, as an equine athlete, is no different. Following a carefully planned training program and timing each period at a particular gait is the best way to avoid the potential for overwork. You must know how long your horse can perform at a trot or canter. Unless you know his or her current abilities, there's no way to determine if you've pushed the limit. If you yourself were on a treadmill, you would know exactly how long you could jog in place without overdoing it. We need to apply the same approach and extend the same consideration to our horses. Overworked muscles become tense muscles and tense muscles can become injured muscles.

Step Three:
Maintaining a Pain and Tension Free Body

Chiropractic and massage type therapies can not only be used to treat existing issues but can also be used in preventing those issues from recurring, or occurring in the first place.

The cause of the joint misalignment, especially if it keeps occurring, must be identified. This discovery will involve a process of elimination, taking many of the topics covered in this book into consideration – shoeing issues, saddle fitting issues, bitting issues, dental issues and rider fitness issues. Any of the above issues, alone or in combination, can contribute to subluxation problems, or cause a re-occurrence until corrected.

Tension Remedies

There are a number of effective ways to identify muscle tension and then release that tension when it occurs. You only have to do a bit of study on the subject to find many helpful suggestions.

One example is Jack Meagher, a pioneer of equine sports massage. He has identified 25 points on a horse's body that he believes to be 'trigger points' to check for muscle tension. In his book, *Beating Muscle Injuries for Horses: 25 Common Muscular Problems, Their Cause, Correction, Prevention,* Meagher explains how to locate those trigger points on your own horse and how to do basic treatment on any tension you find.

Another practitioner who is gaining quick ground in the horse world is Jim Masterson. His *Masterson Method*™ technique of integrated equine therapy is one I highly recommend. He offers a basic, reasonably priced, weekend course on tension release work that every horse owner could benefit from (see recommended resources).

In learning the basics of any massage therapy or tension release work and incorporating it into your horse's daily routine, I think you'll find that it makes a big difference in your own horse's ability to move with ease. Tension free movement makes for a happier and much more cooperative horse.

Once you've identified existing problem areas, any muscle tension concerns you have can be addressed and can start to be relieved by learning the massage therapy techniques mentioned above and by finding an expert in your choice of massage therapy. All horses, no matter if they're used for recreation or for the Olympics, can benefit from muscle tension work. Once tension is developed for any reason, it will stay intact until bodywork is done, as horses cannot release tension themselves.

Keeping It All Together

Many chiropractic or muscle tension issues may require on-going treatment, especially if subluxation or tension has resulted from long-standing conformation challenges created by incorrect shoeing or a bad saddle fit, among others. This highlights the importance of finding a chiropractor/therapist you can put your confidence and trust in as you develop a long-term relationship. With that said, even the work done by the most skilled of chiropractors will quickly become undone if the contributing causes aren't changed, or the horse in question isn't put into a program of appropriate or correct exercise after treatment. Once joints have been realigned, the surrounding muscles must be worked and strengthened correctly in the area to help keep everything in its proper place. If the root of the problem that led to subluxation or muscle tension isn't corrected, the same problem will continue to occur time and time again. Steps must be taken to help your horse stay pain and tension free by doing all you can to eliminate the causes, and to build up their overall strength and condition through proper training.

An Ounce of Prevention...

Many unfortunate situations can be avoided if we take the time to focus on the horse's physiology first. In other words, check out what is going on *under* the saddle before blaming or disciplining the horse. As with every area of consideration covered in the previous and following chapters of this book, it's not my intention to claim "expert" status on the subject or attempt to provide an in-depth answer to every question you may have. My goal is simply to share my own learning experiences and to encourage other horse owners to continue learning for themselves. Finding the people you need to help you through your own challenges becomes much easier as you increase your own knowledge on these subjects. I now rely on my horse Grace's regular chiropractic checks to not only keep her pain free, but also to help me gauge if her conditioning program is correct. I work on tension releases almost daily with Grace and if everything stays in line from one check to the next, I know I'm on the right track in terms of her comfort and conditioning.

Grace's Story

During her stay at a training facility, a chiropractic check for Grace revealed several areas that were in need of adjustment. She had a rib that was out of alignment and twisted, poking her in the side with every move, her left scapula (Fig. 2.7) was

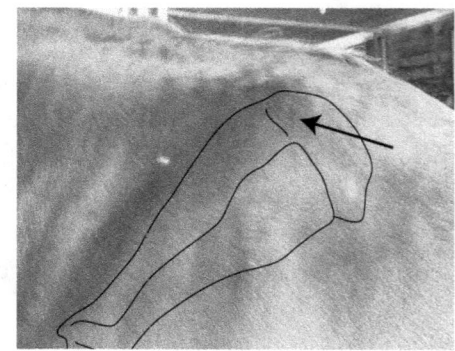

Figure 2.7 Grace's left scapula now corrected.

elevated, her front sesamoids (Fig. 2.8) were locked and her pelvis (Fig. 2.9) was out. The pain must have been bothering her for quite some time. The rib that was out was stabbing her during each breath…*no wonder she didn't want to move out or bend into the right lead.* With hindsight, I realized that a slipping incident in the round pen that occurred a few weeks earlier might have been the root cause of the problem. This taught me quickly how easily a horse can hide pain and how easily it can be overlooked. I now have Grace checked two to four times a year to ensure that everything is in place and as it should be.

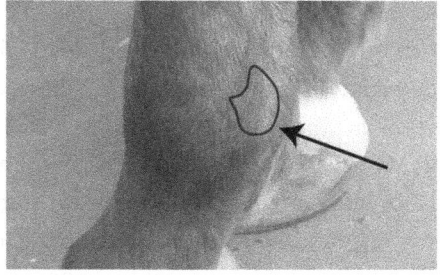

Figure 2.8 The sesmoid area that was locked.

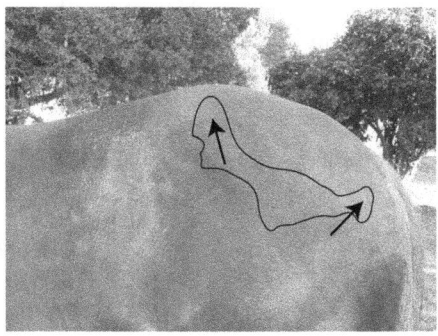

Figure 2.9 The pelvic area now corrected.

After taking a certificate course in the *Masterson Method*™, I became painfully aware that Grace did, in fact, have a lot of tension. This tension was pronounced in her shoulders and front end. It's been a wonderful journey to discover, with great amazement, how much I can help to relieve this for her. There's a new connection developing between us, and it does nothing less than thrill me to think that I can help her to be more comfortable and fluid, not only in her movements, but in her life.

Sound Asleep in the Arena

It was after a good long workout on the lunge line for my horse Grace that I remained in the center of the arena to do a bit of *Masterson Method*™ tension release work on her. She was especially tight in the hind end area on her left. I had noticed this while she was moving. Beginning the release work, I was not only getting the blinks you look for which indicate tension in the horse, but I was getting closed eyes that day. She was really into it! After doing quite a bit of work on releasing her tension, I was done and was ready to exit the arena. As I went to leave, I took a quick glance at her and noticed that she had a bit of a dazed look on her face. Not her usual alert self. I tried again to get her to come with me and still she was not willing to move. She looked to me to 'be in the zone'. As I stood there realizing that she was still processing my work on her, she began that downward perch that horses do when they begin to lay down or roll. Within seconds she had gone down. I started to think that she wanted to roll, but instead she just laid there in that kitty cat position. Mind you there was a lesson going on down at the other end of the arena and other people milling around just outside near us. I decided to go with it and within about a minute; she stretched out completely on her side and just laid there. Someone who was getting her horse ready nearby said: "that's a funny place to take a nap." I chuckled as I thought, "it sure is." Grace proceeded to take a nap for about 10 minute's right there in the arena. Had I not known that it is common for some horses to process this way after tension relief work, I would have wondered what had I done to my horse. A few passers-by asked if she was o.k. and I just said, "She's just sleeping." After a while, someone entered the arena at a gate near us and Grace decided to wake up and we eventually left the arena. I guess the work went well, as the next day she was moving better than ever! For anyone who would love to have a better relationship with their horse, I strongly recommend investigating a weekend course on the *Masterson Method*™.

CHAPTER 3

Understanding Saddle Fitting Basics

Grace's Story

Loping was never Grace's strong suit. She always seemed to labor at that gait. It was an effort for her, even on the lunge line. It also seemed to me that when we attempted it riding, she always "hollowed out" (Fig. 3.1). When transitioning into the lope, she would lift her head and propel herself into the gait. This was confusing to me as she was able to hold her top line so naturally at the trot. I kept getting the feeling that she couldn't control this and wasn't just doing it out of spite. She seemed uncomfortable to me and that made me uncomfortable. I needed to figure out why she propelled herself like that. It dawned on me one day that maybe it was her saddle that was bothering her, so I decided to embark on a mission to learn and understand everything I could about saddle fitting. I studied everything I could get my hands on and even took a certificate course on saddle fitting. After doing a complete inspection of my saddle with the new knowledge I had gained, I discovered my saddle actually didn't fit at all. I had this confirmed again by another professional saddle fitter. I immediately felt horrible at the realization that I had been asking her to comply under an uncomfortable saddle. I have since found a correctly fitted saddle and it's not only obvious that Grace is more comfortable, but she's even more at ease when I approach her to put the saddle on.

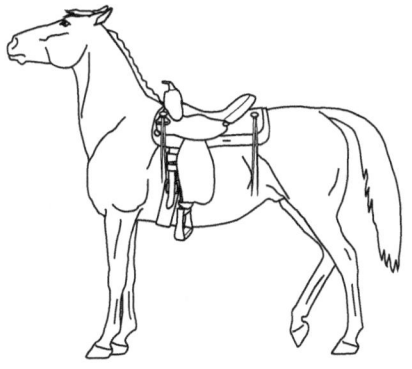

Figure 3.1 Elevated head can mean back pain.

Why Bother?

Whether you ride English or Western, having a saddle that fits is essential to a respectful union with your horse. Proper placement, appropriate weight distribution and the comfort of both horse and rider are all important to achieving the best ride possible. After all, the saddle is one of the main tools we use with the horse. If you've ever worn ill-fitting shoes for any length of time, you'll easily understand what a horse might be experiencing if they were wearing an ill-fitting saddle. It's important to look at saddle fitting with the same detail we might use in choosing our own riding boots. Both need to fit well and be comfortable in order to for us perform to the best of our ability. Sometimes people choose tack based upon a fad color, or because it's on sale. Someone can recommend a saddle they've used with good success on their horse, but each horse is different. Maybe someone is selling a used saddle that they'd love for you to buy. They give it to you to try on your horse and someone says, "Yeah, it looks like it fits." I just want to express that cutting corners in this area can make or break the relationship we have with our horse. It's essential to develop an understanding of your horse's back and the implications of a poor or incorrect choice of saddle.

Ill-Fitting Saddle Behavior
- Anxiety when being saddled.
- Riding with a lifted head and hollow back.
- Not standing still for mounting.
- Tripping.
- Excessive twitching while being groomed.
- Bucking or rearing.
- Unwillingness to go forward; lack of impulsion.
- Reluctance to take a gait or a particular lead in canter.
- Headshaking or pinning of ears.
- Difficulty when shoeing.
- Restlessness when tied up.

Listed above are some of the signs that saddle fit might need to be checked. Your horse may not display every symptom on the list or may not show any symptoms at all. Some horses are very stoic. They've learned to hide their discomfort in order to please, or to avoid discipline. It's worth noting that saddle fit may not be the cause of these behaviors, but it is always good to do a thorough check of your saddle anyway, as it's one of the most important elements of your ride.

If you watch closely, horses can object almost immediately to their saddle, while others may not choose to show resistance. Most of the time, with a little practice and a willingness to pay attention to your horse's mannerisms, you can learn to identify the signs of conflict or of acceptance of a saddle. Evidence of acceptance will be seen in your horse's facial expressions or overall relaxed attitude. Evidence of conflict will be seen in expressions of anxiety, irritation or an overall uptight attitude. This can, or will often result in your horse attempting to move away from the saddle as you place it on his or her back. Sitting on a horse offers us an extension of our own physical capabilities, but how many of us have taken the time to study what lies beneath us and to learn more about what is actually inside the backs of these creatures? (Fig. 3.2)

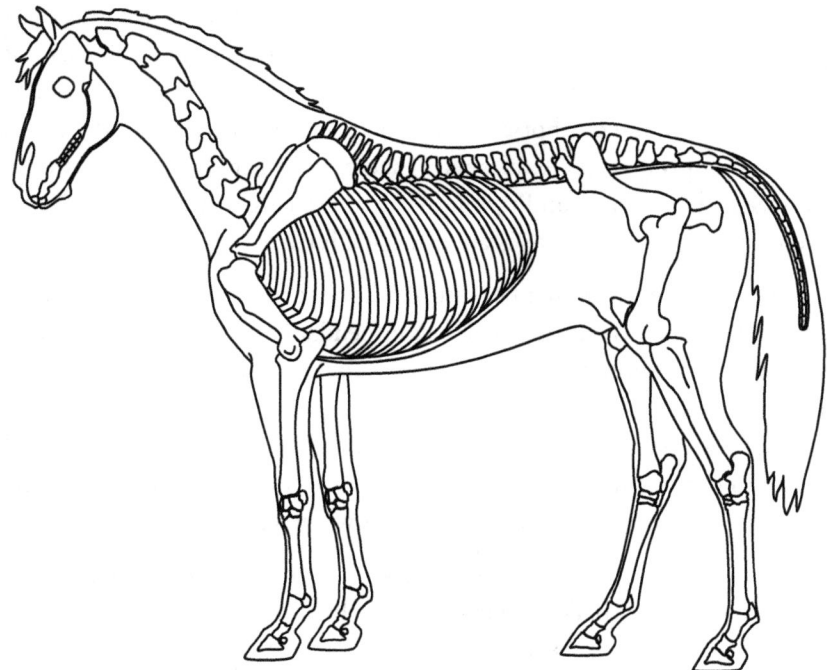

Figure 3.2 The skeletal system of the horse.

What Lies Under Our Saddles?

Along the top of the spine, and therefore directly under where we sit, are a number of sharply pointed bones referred to as the spinous processes (Fig. 3.3). These bones come very close to the surface of the horse's back and are only covered with minimal skin. This means there is great potential for those bones to come into close contact with a saddle, especially once the rider's weight is added. If contact is made with these bones, your horse will experience something similar to that of a pin being pressed up and through a sheet of paper. When you consider the range of complex movements required in the horse's spine to accommodate the variety of maneuvers we expect our horse's to perform, the potential for an ill-fitting saddle to severely limit those movements, or cause pain, becomes clearer with a deeper understanding of what lies beneath. Now take a moment to consider the consequences of an ill-fitting saddle coupled with an unbalanced rider, and think back to the list of "problem" behaviors.

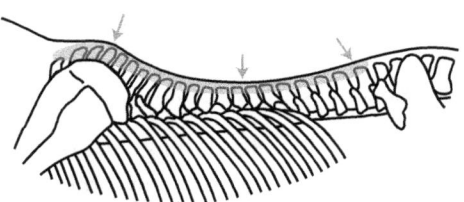

Figure 3.3 Spinous Process: Note how close the bones are to the outer layer of skin on the back. This close proximity of bones to skin can be a real source of pain under an ill-fitting saddle.

UNDERSTANDING SADDLE FITTING BASICS 29

When you find evidence of an ill-fitting saddle you'll probably need the help of an expert saddle fitter with experience in your riding discipline to help you examine your fit. It's also important to remember that things change. Even if you had a saddle fitting done at the time bought your horse, there's no guarantee that your saddle will remain a good fit through the years. A number of factors can generate significant changes, including weight gain or loss, conditioning, structural changes in hoof angles or muscular changes etc.; many of these changes are discussed further in the relevant chapters.

I've heard the justification that because a saddle is of a quality name brand, it must be good for the horse. By all means it's commendable to purchase quality, lifetime tack, but without question, it's not an indication of fit. In my experience, many saddle shops or fitter/sellers have incentives to sell you particular brands or styles. These might be excellent choices, but only if they fit. Someone might benefit from making a sale but it's also possible that you or your horse may not. For this reason, I recommend you always find an independent, impartial fitter whenever possible.

You probably won't get a closer fit than with a custom saddle, but they can be expensive. If cost isn't a challenge for you, then by all means, go for it. Just keep in mind that a made-to-measure saddle will provide a good fit for your horse at the time he or she is measured, but as discussed earlier, measurements can change due to a number of factors. This means that you may end up changing saddles at some point. If you decide to go with a custom saddle, be sure to look for a reputable saddle maker who creates design styles you love.

Other saddle options that people consider include flex or treeless saddles. In my experience, unless a flex saddle fits perfectly, it can become a source of even more pressure or pain. Because it 'flexes' more on a horse's back, it puts more pressure on the limited points of contact if it doesn't fit. Again, if a flex tree fits *near perfect* it can be a good option. Treeless saddles can place all of the pressure of the rider onto one spot on the horse's back. The rider's weight may not be as evenly dispersed across the length of the horse's back muscles as with traditional bars or panels (Fig. 3.4). Again, while I'm sure the flex and treeless saddles have their place in the horse world, I suggest that owners look at well-fitting traditional saddles for the reasons mentioned above.

Saddle fit is a developing area of horsemanship, and I expect new studies and information will continue to become available. For now, one should know that owning a Quarter Horse doesn't necessarily mean you need Quarter horse bars or that if

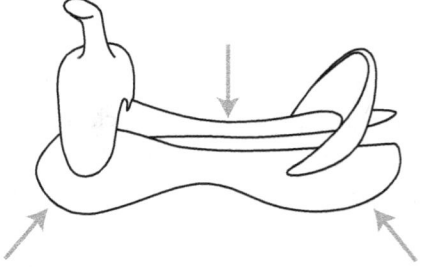

Figure 3.4 Western saddle bars. Weight is dispersed across the entire length of the bars.

you own a Thoroughbred, you need a medium wide tree. The bars are named by the manufactures to serve as a guide to the general buying population, so they are simply a rule of thumb. You still need to check carefully for a correct fit. I recommend that you take advice from the best professionally trained saddle fitter you can find, but even then, educate yourself enough to determine whether the information being provided is correct.

> **BEFORE THE CROP COMES OUT…KEY POINT TO CONSIDER NUMBER 3**
>
> **YOUR HORSE CAN'T MOVE WELL UNDER AN UNCOMFORTABLE SADDLE.**

Basic Parts of the Saddle (figs. 3.5 - 3.8)

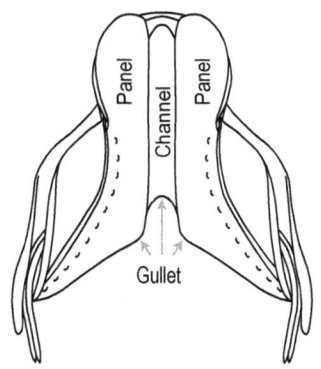

Figure 3.5 Channel and Panels of the saddle.

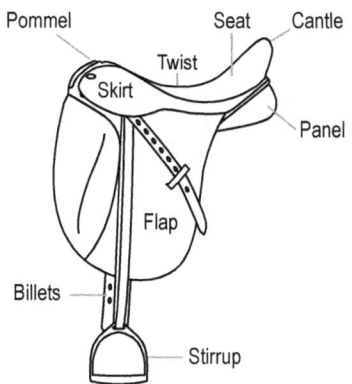

Figure 3.6 Basic Dressage saddle parts.

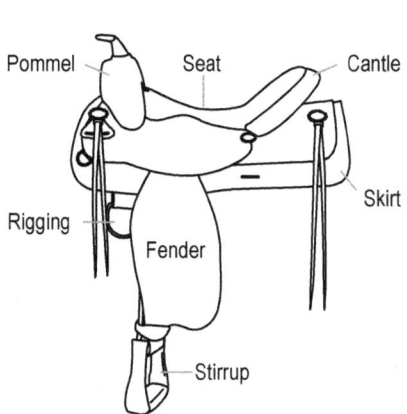

Figure 3.7 Basic Western saddle parts.

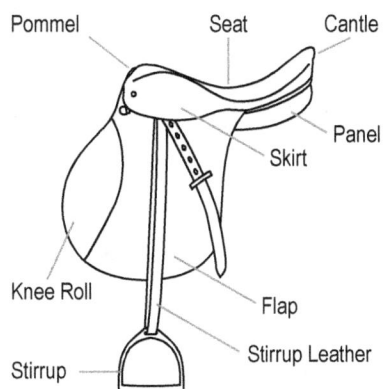

Figure 3.8 Basic English saddle parts.

UNDERSTANDING SADDLE FITTING BASICS 31

How to Check the Saddle Itself

The tree of any saddle can become twisted or broken over time. Make sure that you or a professional fitter check the tree or bars for cracked or broken parts. Place the saddle up-ended on its horn or pommel front end, and apply a substantial amount of downward pressure. Check for any give (Fig. 3.9). The feel should remain rigid (unless it's a flex tree) even when pressure is applied. This should also be the case when checking the amount of side to side give when squeezing the skirting or panels together (Fig. 3.10). It's also important to notice whether the amount of give, or lack of it, feels the same on each side.

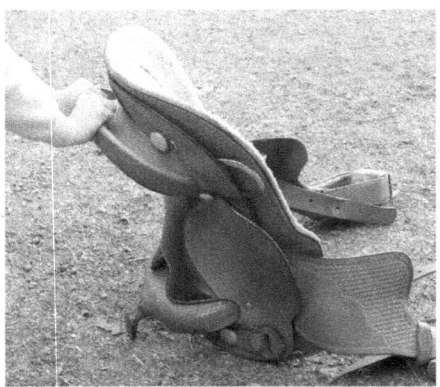

Figure 3.9 Check for give with downward pressure. There should be no give unless the saddle is a flextree. This is applicable for English, Western and Dressage saddles.

New saddles are less likely to have broken trees or bars, but can still have manufacturing defects. In a world of mass-produced machine manufacturing, good quality control is sometimes lacking. The slightest misplacement of a screw or notch can seriously alter the straightness of a saddle. Checking for symmetry is always recommended, even when buying new. To do this, hold the saddle with horn or pommel facing downward and hang it off your right hip if you're right-handed, or off the left hip if you're left-handed. Take a look at the sightline downward toward the ground and see if it appears to be straight (Fig. 3.11).

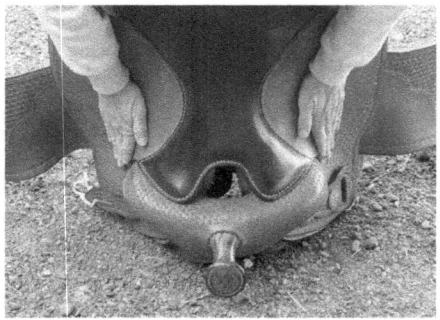

Figure 3.10 Check for any side to side give. The saddle should feel stable.

From this angle, it becomes easier to check for any asymmetry or imbalance. Further checks include fender alignment and stirrup alignment. These can be done from above using a saddle tree, or can be done on the ground. Pull out the fenders and stirrups to view any imperfections or offsets and then turn the saddle over to check for even wear on both sides underneath; all things should appear even and balanced (Fig. 3.12).

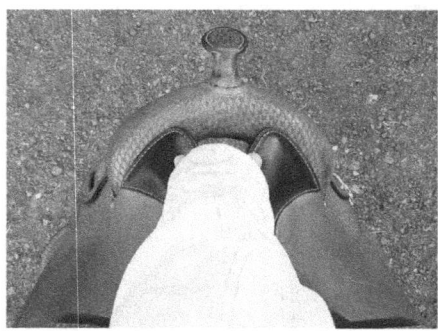

Figure 3.11 Check for evenness using a sight line off the hip of your holding hand. Look for any asymmetry or unbalance. Manufacturing flaws can be seen in this position as well as on a saddle rack from above.

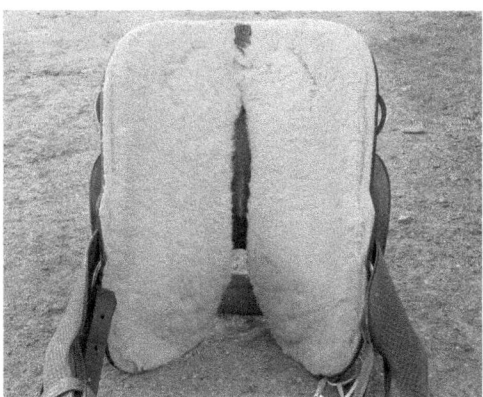

Figure 3.12 View the saddle from underneath. Look for balance in either the wear of the sheepskin on a Western saddle or in the stuffing of the panels on an English or Dressage saddle. Minor differences can make a big difference to the horse.

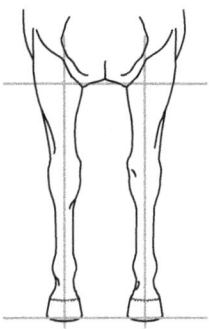

Figure 3.13 Front leg picture frame. Make sure that there are no initial changes needed in shoeing. These changes will need to be made before getting a good saddle fit.

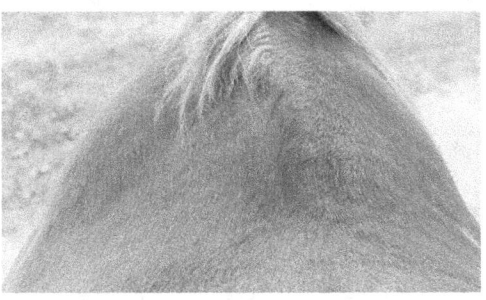

Figure 3.14 Compare of the shoulder area from a high rear view from behind the horse. Be careful that you and your horse are safe in this position.

Things to Look For Before Fitting

These basic checks should be done without any saddle padding, with the horse standing on the most level ground possible and squared up with all four feet.

- **From the front:**

  Look for symmetry in the front leg picture frame area (Fig. 3.13); this is similar when looking at shoeing angles. Unless this area is symmetrical, all other measurements can be off.

- **From the rear:**

  Is there an elevated shoulder height (Fig. 3.14) on one side or the other? Asymmetry in the horse's shoulders leads to the saddle constantly shifting forwards on the elevated side. This is an issue that will require corrected shoeing and time to remedy. There are some pad modifications that can be done by scooping out the area near the larger shoulder, but this requires a bit of careful work to be done correctly.

- **From above (positioning yourself on a short riser):**

  Palpate the back on both sides of the spine from the pocket area, two inches behind the shoulders, all the way back to the loin area. This should be done using your fingertips on the area of the back where the saddle would sit above the ribcage (Fig. 3.15). Check for signs of pain or discomfort in the muscles. However, in determining whether your horse is showing signs of pain,

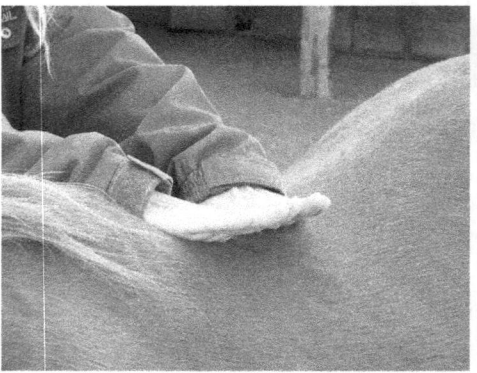 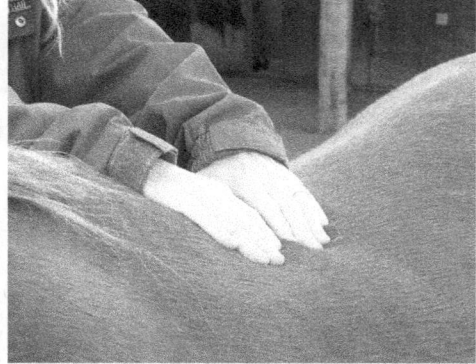

Figure 3.15 Palpate the back, using a riser, standing on the side. Assess if there are tender spots or any soreness where the bars or panels have made contact with the back.

it must be remembered that the muscles will naturally be more delicate if you ride infrequently. This can be likened to walking barefoot; the more often you do it, the less sensitive the soles of your feet become. For this reason, it would be best not to check for signs of discomfort the day after a ride unless your horse is accustomed to a similar level of activity on a regular basis. If your horse has been ridden regularly, any signs of wincing or shifting as you palpate the muscles will give you a pretty good indication of where sore spots may already exist.

Check List for Good Basic Fit

- **Do you have the saddle in the natural pocket of the horse?**

  This is accomplished by placing the saddle well in front of the withers and then sliding it back until it comes to a natural resting place, or its home. Sliding the saddle backward in this way is a much more accurate way of determining the correct position compared to the more common practice of placing the saddle directly onto the horses back from the side where we think it should go. Where the saddle lies naturally will vary based on fit, but each saddle must be put in its natural place first as all other checks can only be made accurately after this placement—it will end up in its natural resting place after a while anyway as it works its way there, no matter where you place it to begin with (Fig. 3.16).

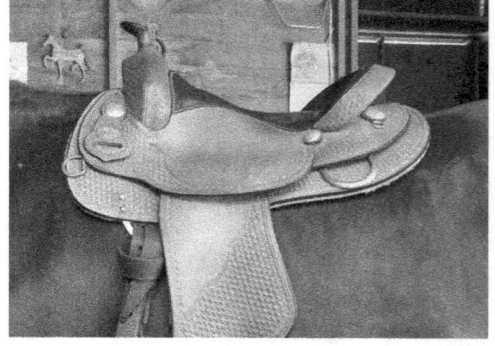

Figure 3.16 Find the natural resting place of the saddle.

- **Is there enough room for the withers?**

  Once the saddle is positioned in the natural pocket, you must check to see if there's enough room for your horse's withers from all angles, and down through the gullet backward as far as you can feel (Fig. 3.17). This can be accomplished by using the feel of your hand, reaching inside the front of the saddle to check the area all along the withers, including the rear of the withers. Horses with tight fitting saddles in this area can be in great pain. Just use common sense to consider the consequences for the structurally large wither bones positioned here. Placing a riding crop or other similar straight object down through the channel of the saddle will also help determine space. There should be ample clearance down and through. Using a stool and a flashlight can help you to view down and inside this area. This light can also help you to see possible bridging (explained further below).

- **Is the saddle sitting level on the horse?**

  This is something that can be deceiving, so be prepared to develop an eye through practice. A more accurate assessment can be made by looking at cantle and pommel height differences as opposed to looking at differences in the skirting levels or fenders (Fig. 3.18).

- **Do the angles of the bars in front match the angle of your horse's shoulder muscles?**

  This is best determined by looking from the front and running your hand, with palm up, from the top of the bar

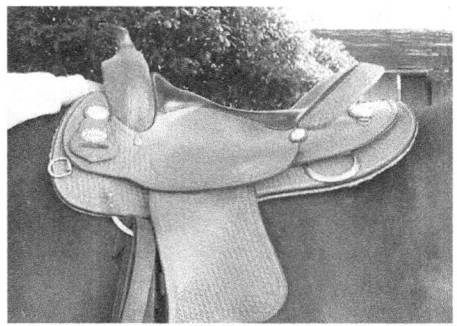

Figure 3.17 Using your hand, reach down through the pommel and feel as far back as you can. Check for any contact with the withers or any tightness in that area.

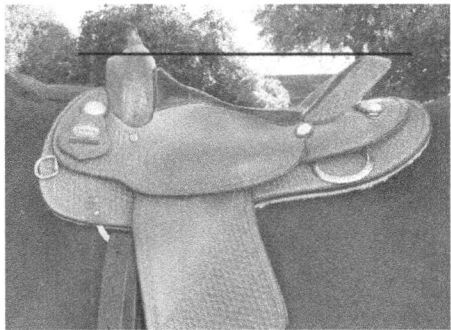

Figure 3.18 Check for levelness of the pommel and cantle of the saddle instead of looking at the skirting which can sometimes be deceiving.

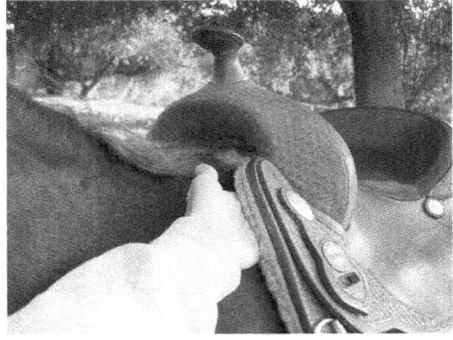

Figure 3.19 Palm side up, check from the top of the bars or points to the bottom of the bars or points for tightness, looseness or pinching. It is a good idea to also check this while walking the horse in a circle.

or point down to the bottom. There should be even contact all the way down with no evidence of pinching or pressure (Fig. 3.19). This should be done on both sides.

- **Do the panels or bars make even contact all along your horses back?**

Another common fitting issue is bridging. This is when the four points of the bars in a Western saddle, or the four corners of the panels in an English or Dressage saddle, are the only points underneath that make contact with the horse's back (Fig. 3.20). The remaining area makes no connection with the rest of the back muscles. This creates uneven weight distribution across the bars or panels, focuses all of the saddle and rider's weight on just four points, and should be avoided. Without balanced and even distribution, the concentrated pressure can be enough to cut off the blood supply to the muscles in the areas of pressure. This can cause dead muscle tissue or atrophy, and happens quickly. Once destroyed, the tissue will never come back to life.

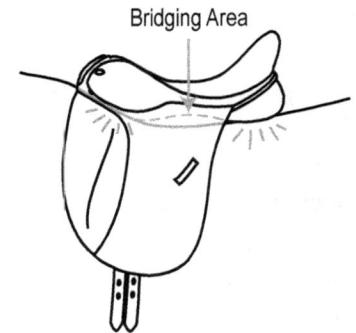

Figure 3.20 Example of a saddle that is bridging. Notice the lack of contact in the middle area.

On an English or Dressage saddle, re-flocking can sometimes help to establish a correct fit, but not in every case. There must be a close fit to begin with for re-flocking to be effective. Western saddles are a bit more critical, as the bars underneath cannot be changed. On a Western saddle, it's not uncommon for riders or fitters to use pads in an effort to fill this bridged or ill-fitting area. It can be very difficult to check for bridging in a Western saddle, with the weight of the extra leather complicating matters. Like the story of the princess and the pea, the horse can feel the rise and fall of everything, so unless pads are *carefully* constructed with very smooth tapers, this just becomes another source of irritation or pain. I recommend that any bridging adjustments, if done at all, be done by a reputable and caring professional. Unless there's a fairly good fit to begin with, it's always best to move on and try a different saddle.

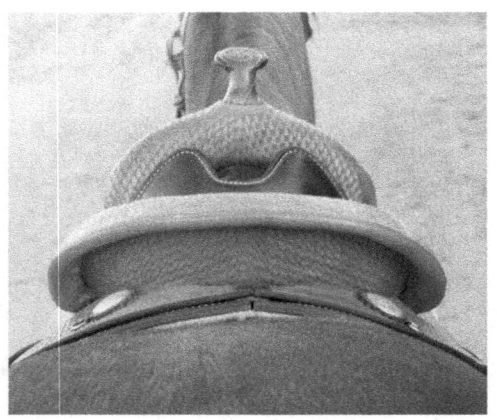

Figure 3.21 Look for nice even contact in the loin area. A small gap between the horse and the skirting on a western saddle is recommended. On an English or Dressage saddle, look for perching or riding on the inside edges of the panels.

- **Do the angles of the panels or bars match the angles of your horse's loin area?**

  This is best seen from the rear (Fig. 3.21). A saddle that's too wide will make contact with a horse's back on the inner edges but not the outer, and a saddle that's too narrow will appear to perch on the horse's back, making contact only on the outer edges. Also check to see if the panels or bars are even.

- **Does the saddle rock on the horse?**

  Too much forward and backward movement or rocking of the saddle indicates that there are fitting issues and the saddle is potentially too wide (Fig. 3.22a and Fig 3.22b). Using a pad or a series of pads may help to *adjust* the fit of a saddle, but the bottom line will always be that a pad can't *"fix"* an ill-fitting saddle. If a saddle is too small, a larger pad will not prevent it from pinching, just as wearing larger socks will not ease your pain if your shoes are too small. The same applies to using extra padding when a saddle is too large; the end result is more than likely an unsteady saddle. There have been times when a particular pad used has helped a saddle to fit better, but this is more the exception than the rule.

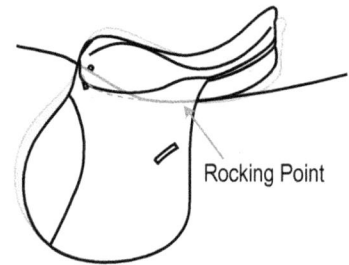

Figure 3.22a Understanding rocking

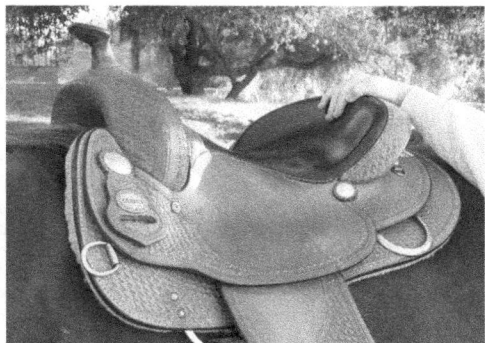

Figure 3.22b Checking for rocking

- **Is the saddle centered over the ribcage of the horse?**

  In order to check this carefully, it may be helpful to refer to the earlier skeletal illustration. Locate the position of your horse's last rib by feeling along his or her ribcage with your hand, then find the pocket (the deepened area located about two inches behind the shoulder). This is your horse's full rib cage. The saddle should sit in the middle of this area (Fig. 3.23).

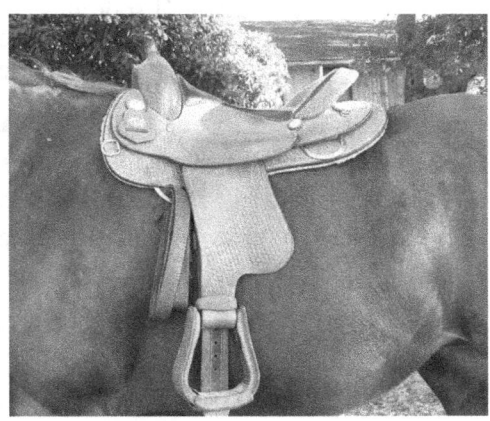

Figure 3.23 View the horse from the side to see if the saddle fits over the center of the rib cage. Feel with your hand for the last rib. This will help you determine if it is sitting too far back.

- **Is the saddle too long?**

  It's possible for a saddle to be too long for a horse's back. When your saddle is positioned correctly in its home, the bars or panels shouldn't extend beyond your horse's last rib. If the length extends past this point, your saddle is sitting over the loin area, which can't support the weight of a saddle, let alone a rider as well; and if the skirting is too long, as in a Western saddle, it will hit your horse in the hip with every stride (Fig. 3.24).

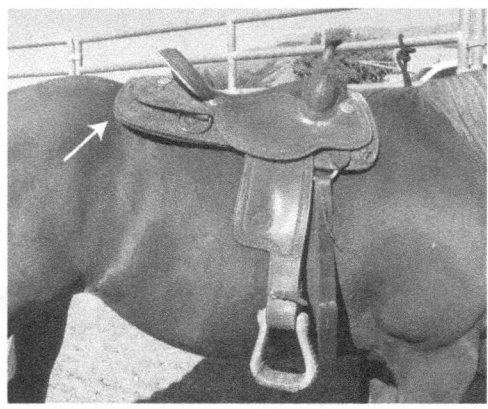

Figure 3.24 Look for the skirt to see if it is making contact with the hip of the horse. As you can see, this saddle is too long for the back of this horse.

- **Does the center of the seat meet with the center of your horse's back?**

  The center of the seat of the saddle—where your legs would naturally hang—should meet with the center of your horse's back. This can be measured using a simple 3-inch level available in most hardware stores. Identify the lowest point on your horse's back, find the level spot and mark the location with a sticker or a temporary mark of some sort on the

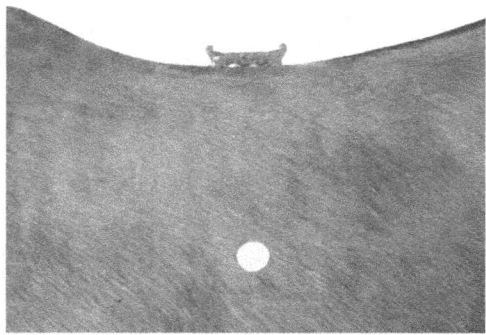

Figure 3.25 Find the low and level point on the horse's back with a small level purchased at many hardware stores. Mark the spot in line with the level on the side of the horse with a sticky dot or other mark.

horse's side (Fig. 3.25). Now place the saddle in its natural pocket and identify the lowest level point of the saddle in the same way. The two locations should be in close alignment (Fig. 3.26). This applies to all saddle types, Western, English or Dressage, and to every style in each category.

- **What does the sweat pattern tell you?**

  Another quick way to make a general assessment is to look at the saddle's sweat patterns on the horse's back following a ride or a workout. Look for even wetness from the front to the back with no dry areas over the muscles where the bars or panels lie. Dry areas show signs of pressure except along the spine where the channel of the saddle doesn't make contact. If you use a white riding pad, the dirt marks on the underside of the pad can read like a map showing tell-tale signs of uneven contact. This is another good way to assess pressure, or lack of it, in various areas.

If all of the basic fitting points check out, the next step is to work through the checklist again with a rider in the saddle. Areas that appeared to be fine from the initial check may not be once a rider is in the saddle. Rider fit is also important. There's no point in continuing to check the fit on your horse if the saddle is too small or too big for you.

Rider Fit

Saddle seats that are too small or too large will constantly put you, the rider, out of the correct position. You will inevitably end up fighting with that saddle until you buy another. Don't get hung up on seat size, all manufactures specifications can be different in this area. This is actually a hip to knee measurement. The most important thing is to make sure that you feel balanced and comfortable; you may need an onlooker to view you or take pictures or video from the front, rear and sides to assess how centered and balanced you are in the seat. These pictures or shots will be good for you to see as well.

Final Notes on Fitting

Fitting challenges in English or Dressage saddles are typically pretty easy to spot. Because Western saddles can be a bit more difficult, I've found it helpful to use a set of 'Equi-fit® Fit To Be Seen®' fiberglass forms (Fig. 3.27) made by Steele Saddle Tree LLC (see recommended resources). These are designed to simulate the bars of a Western saddle. The nine different forms look amazingly similar lying side by side, yet on the horse can look drastically different. Considering the

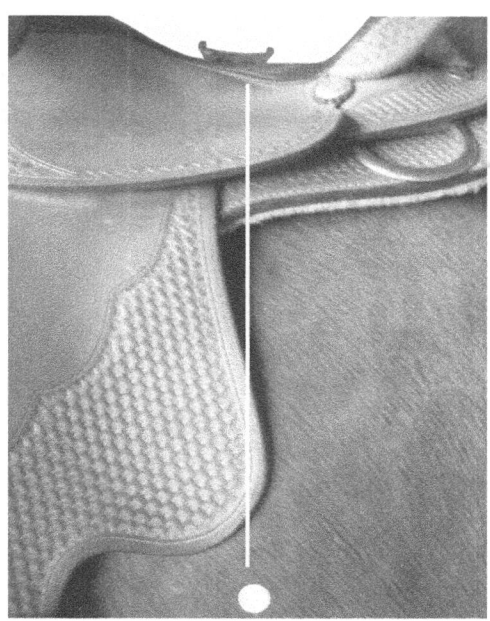

Figure 3.26 After placing the saddle on your horse, find the low and level spot on the saddle. The sticky dot and the level now on the saddle should be in close alignment.

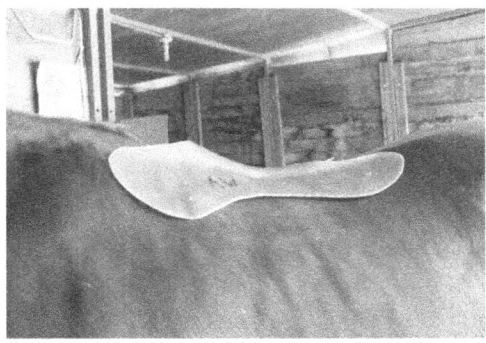

Figure 3.27 A Steel Saddle Tree Fit Form. With these forms you or a fitter can make a clear observation as to fit. These are made in replica for the bars in some western saddles currently for sale.

25 pounds or so of weight on a Western saddle, it's extremely important to be able to recognize the telltale signs of acceptance or conflict.

There's no such thing as a perfect saddle fit, but you owe it to yourself and your horse to get the best fit you can. Again, I recommend consulting with a reputable professional. An experienced and *intuitive* saddle fitter can be vital, and should be included on your team.

It troubles me greatly how easily and often a horse's discomfort is overlooked and dismissed as bad behavior. Owners can become so disappointed and disillusioned that they end up selling or giving their horse away, all for the lack of proper information. Many a rejected "problem" horse might have simply been reacting to an ill-fitting saddle.

CHAPTER 4

Bit Choice and Bit Resistance

After discovering that my horse's saddle didn't fit, I began to wonder what else might be contributing to discomfort for her. In pursuit of further knowledge and understanding of what might cause pain in horses, I found a lot of good information on bits. In learning about bits and bit fitting, I discovered that my bits did not fit my horse, either. Not only were they too narrow, they were also too severe for her age and level of training. I began to search the information to learn all I could about bits and how they work, and quickly became convinced that this might be *the* most undiscovered source of riding problems today. I explored this education for my own horse's sake, but now I notice bit resistance with other horses all the time. Here is some basic information to help you get started on your own voyage of discovery. Again, as with your choice of saddles, the goal is a relaxed and accepting attitude from your horse towards your choice of bit.

What Might Be Wrong With Our Bit Choice?

Bits are often a source of misunderstanding in the horse world. I don't know if the problem stems from years of misapplied names or our tendency to stick with the bits we've known since childhood. It might be a lack of understanding of the device in the first place, but it seems that we can forget to consider how a bit actually works, or why we even chose the one we use. It could be that your present choice of a bit is simply a "traditional" choice based on nothing more than the fact that it's a bit you've used for years and on all of your other horses. Unfortunately, your traditional choice may not be the best choice for your current horse. It's my experience, from watching horse after horse and seeing countless signs of bit resistance that we need to take a fresh look at how we make our bit choices. Maybe your choice was based on the recommendation of a trainer or riding instructor, or the opinion of someone working in a tack shop, but I have to ask the difficult question: are these sources really experts on bits? Not always. I've often seen high-level horses, in training, under the watchful eyes of one or more trainers, being ridden in bits too narrow for them, and with obvious resistance. Some of these bits, I'm sure, have been used for years without notice. The bottom line is that horses, just like people, are individuals and the type of bit that worked well for another of your horses, or someone else's horse, isn't necessarily the correct type for your current or future horse. Without careful consideration and some real education in this area, we may be forcing our horses into a very uncomfortable situation, again, sacrificing physical capabilities, our best communication and our relationship.

I've discovered that many people in the horse industry don't have a clear understanding of what bit they use and why. I value the fact that there are many approaches to bits, and respect a well-explained method for choosing one if it makes good common sense. In this chapter, though, I want to elaborate on the most common misunderstandings I've learned about concerning bits. One of the biggest challenges is perhaps the simple fact that there are just too many choices available. There is a vast array of bits available in tack shops or online. Understanding the function of each one can be difficult, but not impossible. First of all, I'm a firm believer in buying bits in person. It's hard to buy something unknown without a feel for it. Does it pinch? Does the balance feel good in your hand? These explorations aren't possible without hands-on testing. We often make a bit choice based on style or cost without taking into consideration the fact that the bit is a critical piece of equipment, especially when it comes to communication with our equine partners. When faced with so many varieties to choose from, it's only natural that you would look to others for help and advice, but not all equine "experts" are bit fitting experts. Once again, I'm not suggesting for a moment that there is a complete lack of education out there about bits, but knowing the name of a bit doesn't equate to understanding how it works in your horse's mouth. What level of training does your horse have? Are you buying the bit for the reaction it will generate? I urge you to research your current choice for your own horse. The more we know as riders or owners, the more we're able to prevent our horses from experiencing discomfort. The more we know, the less likely we are to unwittingly contribute to any unnecessary conflict, discomfort or pain. The purpose of this chapter is not to make you an instant expert, but to make you more aware of the questions you may need to ask of those who are in a position to influence your choices.

Snaffle Bit verses Curb Bit: What's the difference?
- **A snaffle bit is a direct pressure bit.** (Fig. 4.1)

   The principle behind a snaffle bit is that its action is engaged directly by the pull of the rider's hands. As the rider, you are controlling your horse by creating direct pressure on his or her mouth, bars, lips and tongue when you pull on the reins (one pound of rein pressure created by your hands is equal to one pound of pressure on your horse's mouth). **There is no poll or chin groove pressure with a snaffle** and this type of bit is typically used on an untrained or green horse and in the English and Dressage disciplines. These bits help place the horse, or a portion of the horse, where you want them. Direct pressure on the mouth can help to keep a horse in check until advanced training allows them to move into a more yielding bit with more relief. Youngsters or green horses typically need a bit with a tad more 'bite' to establish an initial firm connection until further training teaches them how to work more through seat and leg aids and less through direct pressure. The same would be the case with a lower level English or Dressage horse until further advanced training is achieved.

Important note: A common example of a direct pressure bit is the simple, jointed snaffle. The term "snaffle" is often incorrectly used in relation to any bit with a broken mouthpiece. This can be confusing. However, not all snaffles have a broken mouthpiece and not all bits with a broken mouthpiece are direct pressure bits or snaffles. This highlights the importance of understanding the action of a bit, not just knowing its name.

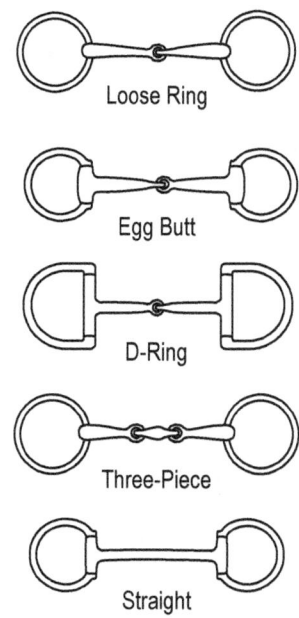

Figure 4.1 Some examples of snaffle bits.

- **A curb bit is an indirect pressure bit.** (Fig. 4.2)

    With this type of bit, there is **both poll *and* chin groove pressure**. Reins are attached to shanks and it's the shanks, no matter how long or short, that create a leverage system through which pressure can be applied indirectly to the horse's mouth, poll and chin by the pull of the rider's hands. These bits are used on horses that have reached a level of training that allows them to know what you are asking of them and understand how to respond after being asked. They aren't used to *increase* pressure on the mouth, but to *decrease* it. Horses that are ready for these bits already know and understand about the positioning of their shoulders, for example, and respond to seat and leg aids.

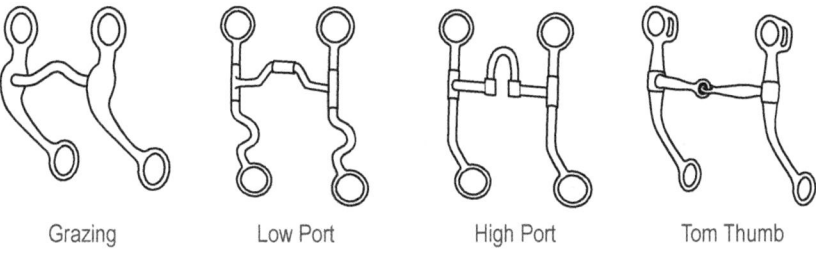

Figure 4.2 Some examples of curb bits.

BIT CHOICE AND BIT RESISTANCE   43

*SHANK RATIO = **the length of the shank to which the reins are attached below the mouthpiece, divided by the length of the shank above the mouthpiece, also known as the purchase.*** (Fig. 4.3)

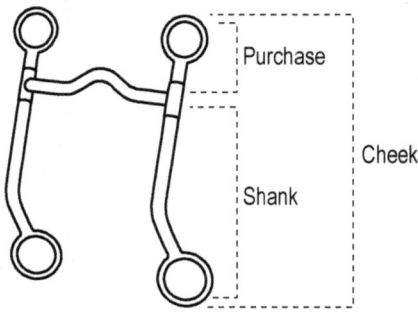

Figure 4.3 Shank ratio.

The length of the shank dictates the force of the pressure. One pound of rein pressure generated by your hands becomes significantly greater than one pound of pressure in your horse's mouth. The longer the shank is, the greater the ratio is. The greater the ratio is, the greater the pressure experienced by your horse at the slightest touch. For example, if the length of shank below the mouthpiece is three inches and the length above (or purchase) is one inch, your bit has a shank ratio of 3:1, (see Fig. 4.3) meaning the 10 pounds of rein pressure you apply with your hands will be experienced as 30 pounds of pressure by your horse. For this reason, it's extremely important for the shank ratio to be appropriate for the skill level of the rider; the less experienced the hands, the smaller the shank ratio should be. Unfortunately, bigger or more severe bits are sometimes used to replace good horsemanship. This should never be the case.

Bit Mouthpieces

The huge variety of bits available to choose from is made even more bewildering by the vast number of different mouthpieces found on each variety. Again, a snaffle can have a straight mouthpiece or a broken mouthpiece, and the break can be a single joint, double joint or more. A curb may also have either a broken or solid mouthpiece. Pressure created by a straight mouthpiece is less severe than that created by the nutcracker action of a broken mouthpiece. Of course, the ideal bit isn't necessarily the one you're most attracted to in the tack shop. Finding the ideal bit for your horse requires understanding the shape of his or her mouth, the level of training of both horse and rider, and finally, your horse's acceptance of it.

Common Bit Resistance Issues

Note: The common behavioral symptoms of bit resistance could mirror results of an ill-fitting saddle, underlying shoeing issues or dental problems, so it's important to rule out or remedy these issues with appropriate checks before directing your focus solely onto your bit or vice versa.

- **Inverting or going above the bit:** (Fig. 4.4)
  This is seen when engaging your reins and describes the head lifting action your horse takes in an effort to move the bit further back in his or her mouth momentarily to be able to swallow.

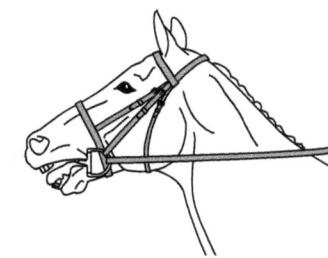

Figure 4.4 Inverting.

- **Going behind the bit:** (Fig. 4.5)
  This is the action your horse takes to tuck his or her head in to such a degree that you effectively lose control and need to release the reins to remedy the situation. In so doing, you inadvertently have allowed your horse momentary relief to be able to swallow.

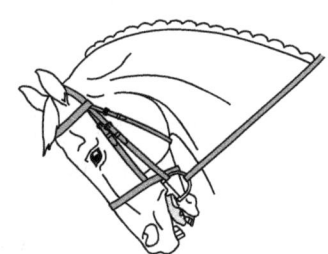

Figure 4.5 Going behind the bit.

- **Getting heavy or rooting:** (Fig. 4.6)
  Depending on the amount of resistance, this can rapidly become a pulling war between you and your horse. In most cases, your horse will eventually pull the reins from your hands, pulling you off balance in the process. Again, this gives your horse a brief moment to recover some relief while you reposition yourself in the saddle.

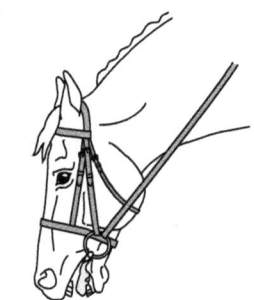

Figure 4.6 Getting heavy or rooting.

- **Gapping or chewing excessively:** (Fig. 4.7)
  This behavior is indicative of a horse's anxiety and overall worrisome condition concerning the bit. By chewing excessively, your horse is expressing discomfort, resulting in resistance and an inability to relax and accept the bit.

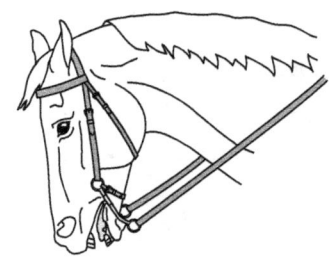

Figure 4.7 Gapping or Chewing excessively.

- **Tongue out of mouth:** (Fig. 4.8)
  If your horse has resorted to sticking their tongue out of their mouth, there is every chance that they've tried to communicate their discomfort in other ways for some time, but now find this compromising action to be the only way of finding relief.

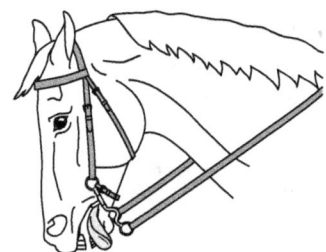

Figure 4.8 Tongue out of the mouth.

- **Tongue over bit:** (Fig. 4.9)
  Similar to sticking out their tongue, your horse may resort to putting his or her tongue over the bit as a more advanced sign of resistance, again, often the result of having tried to communicate their challenges in other ways over a period of time.

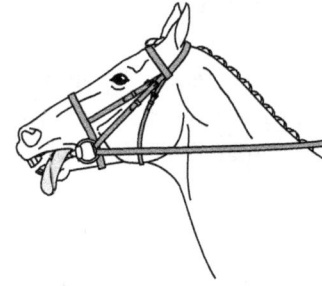

Figure 4.9 Tongue over the bit

- **Drawing tongue into the mouth:** (Fig. 4.10)
  This is another advanced resistance tactic used by your horse in an effort to find relief.

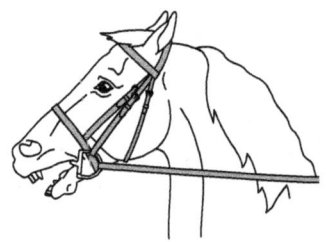

Figure 4.10 Drawing tongue into mouth.

With a keen eye and an open heart, you can help your horse by making the correct decision when choosing a bit; all you have to do is take the time to look for the various signs that will alert you to your horse's concerns. Video can be very helpful for you to see possible resistance issues yourself.

> **BEFORE THE CROP COMES OUT…KEY POINT TO CONSIDER NUMBER 4**
>
> **CHECK YOUR BIT. YOUR HORSE CAN'T TELL YOU IF IT'S UNCOMFORTABLE BUT THEIR BEHAVIOR CAN.**

Understanding the Mouth

A basic mouth check allows you to assess the overall space available in your horse's mouth to accommodate a bit, especially those kinder, fatter bits. The areas to pay particular attention to are the width of the mouth, the tongue and the palate.

Bit Width Sizing

Bits come in different sizes, so an essential element of choosing the correct size of bit for your horse is to measure the exact width of his or her mouth. To do this accurately, you will need a piece of string, a dowel or a bit measuring devise.

- If using a string or dowel, mark one end with a pen or tape. Stand on the left side of your horse and place it inside their mouth as you would a bit, holding the mark in your fingers in your right hand and lining it up with the far side of the mouth to identify your starting point of measurement.

- With the string or dowel comfortably positioned through the mouth and over the tongue, place a mark or hold the measuring devise to identify your second point of measurement on the near side of the mouth. (Fig. 4.11)

- Remove the string, dowel or measuring devise to calculate the distance between the two marks and record the exact width of your horse's mouth. If the measurement is between bit sizing differences, round up. It may take a few tries before your horse stops chewing and moving, allowing you to get a good measurement.

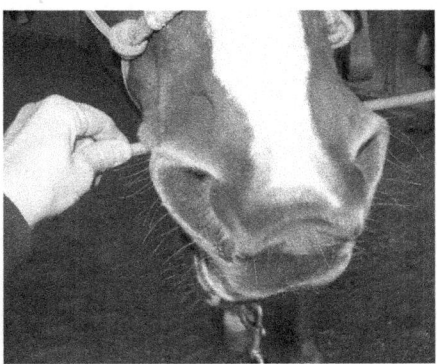

Figure 4.11 Using a string, dowel or the recommended bit measuring device, wait until the horse stops chewing to get a good measurement. You can do this a few times to get an average.

- If fitting a solid mouthpiece, this measurement will be the actual distance between both marks. If fitting a broken mouthpiece, add at least 1/8 inch to both sides for a correct fit.

There is a good measuring device on the market called 'The Original BitFit® – equine mouth measurement tool.' It's easy to use and reasonably priced (see recommended resources).

Once you've identified the correct bit width for your horse, it's also important to identify the correct mouthpiece thickness. A wider, therefore kinder bit may be your first choice, but be sure to check and see if it allows enough room for the horse's tongue. That brings us to the subject of understanding the space inside the mouth.

Tongue – a large tongue will obviously leave less space available for the bit. A simple way to check is to part your horse's lips while his or her mouth is still closed and look for signs of the tongue bulging out over the bars. If it does show bulging over the bars, he or she has a large tongue. As a general rule, the mouthpiece should fill no more than half the space available between the palate and the bars – the fleshy area on the lower jaw between the front and back teeth. (Fig. 4.12)

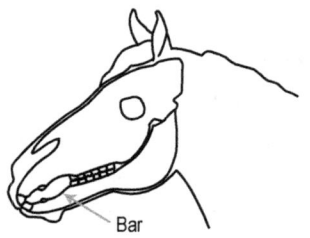

Figure 4.12 The bar area is where you look inside the horse's mouth for a protruding tongue.

Palate – the shape or height of your horse's palate will not only affect the amount of overall space available but also the amount of room available to accommodate different bit actions. The shape of the palate can be assessed by putting an index finger, with the knuckle up, inside at the bar area where a bit would go. When the horse stops chewing, bend your finger. If it touches the roof of the mouth, he or she has a low palate. (Fig. 4.13)

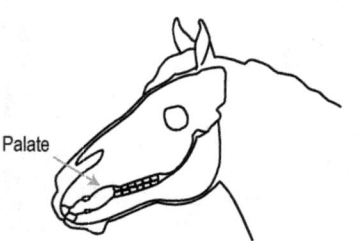

Figure 4.13 The finger goes in straight, palm down, with the knuckle facing upwards; bend the finger to see if it hits the palate. If it does, you have a low palate.

Common Misconceptions and Next Steps

Now that you understand basic fit, it's important to discuss bit mouthpieces once again. Many folks use a simple jointed snaffle in the mistaken belief that they're using a mild bit on their horse. In fact, this couldn't be further from the truth. The nutcracker effect of a single-jointed mouthpiece makes it one of the most severe mouthpieces you can use. Another truth is that these bits prohibit the ability of the horse to swallow correctly. If you're in doubt, place your own finger across your tongue and try to swallow; I think you'll find the results interesting. The ability to swallow not only affects the horse psychologically but affects them physically too. The tongue is attached to the neck, shoulders and sternum muscles that have a direct impact on collection, performance and tension. A horse that is unable to swallow can't perform at his or her best.

I've heard the argument that a single-jointed snaffle is *severe* because it hits the roof of the mouth when rein pressure is applied. If you play with a headstall attached to one of these bits and pull the reins back, the bit collapses forward, not up. This "severity issue" over the single-jointed snaffle is more about the nutcracker effect than a palate hitting issue. Some of the bits on the market today demonstrate a new understanding for tongue relief and its benefit to the horse. There's more information available on this subject, and I recommend that you do your own research. Again, a full examination of all details will give you a better picture of what you need.

> ***Rides are so much better when the horse can actually swallow.***

It's not difficult to imagine how much better we could make things for our horses if we consider how we ourselves would feel if we had to run for any distance without being able to swallow correctly.

If, when checking your horse's mouth, you discover signs of damage caused by a poorly fitted or inappropriate bit, you may need to begin your search for the ideal bit by using the *mildest* bit feasible. Consider and address any rider issues that may have played a part. It's good to note here that there are bits that not only use points of the mouth to communicate, but also use subtle nose and poll pressure to guide the horse into softness. These can help horses that may have been previously hurt, or are in need of relief, to start over.

A Change in the Industry

I've heard estimates by a number of bit experts that as many as 80 to 90 percent of horses with problem behavior have issues with an incorrect bit. Such behavior can be anything from a lack of simple softening to outright refusal to move forward. A change in bit choice or size can sometimes radically affect a horse's willingness to respond correctly. The challenge at present is not only the lack of bit knowledge in the industry, but also that mass-production manufacturers here and abroad typically only want to produce the standard 5-inch or few common sizes in most styles. This is in part because of demand and because of production costs. It's good to know that there *are* bit makers that will customize bits to any specific size. It's advisable to search them out if your horse's measurements don't match the standard sizes. Custom bits might cost more upfront, but in the long run, money spent on riding lessons or training, trying to accomplish what a simple bit change can, will far outweigh the cost of the right bit. It's imperative to have the proper device for our horses' comfort and physical longevity.

Bit fitting is a process of discovery. Again, I recommend that you find a trained bit fitter or consultant. You only need to care enough to take the time to watch and explore this small but fundamental issue about your horse to make a huge difference in his or her world.

CHAPTER 5

Nutrition and Dental

Grace's Feeding Story

Most boarding facilities in my area feed twice a day, morning and evening. Because I was usually at the stable only in the middle of the day, I never actually saw the horses being fed. One day I arrived early for a ride and noticed that the horses hadn't been fed yet, and they seemed uncomfortable about it. So, on mornings that I arrived early, I began to check whether or not the horses were fed. Sometimes they were, sometimes they weren't. I couldn't help feeling that this must be hard on them. When I moved to a facility where the horses were consistently fed at the same time each day, I realized how much more peaceful the horses seemed overall. After studying nutrition and the horse's digestive system, I'm convinced that frequent feedings, and in sufficient amounts, will help to increase a horse's comfort and reduce anxiety.

The Big Picture

The subject of diet and nutrition for horses (or humans) can be very daunting and confusing. It's not my intention to attempt to cover every aspect of equine nutrition in one short chapter, but simply to draw attention to the fact that it is one more area of horse care that needs careful consideration.

The Natural Digestive Design

Horses have relatively small stomachs. They're naturally designed to graze continuously throughout the day, eating small amounts over a long period of time. Left on their own, they can graze for 16-18 hours a day. In the wild, grazing horses are continually on the move, and this, along with the high fiber content of natural forage, helps to promote a healthy gut by aiding the passage of food through the digestive system. A horse will also drink an average of 12 gallons of water in a day, following the same "little and often" principle. Domestic or stabled horses are commonly fed just twice a day. This type of schedule, for the kept horse, leaves the digestive tract empty for a long time. Lack of food in the system, along with limited daily movement in stalls, can lead to ulcers, colic and other serious digestive issues. It's important for the comfort and the health of our horses to pay attention to their natural design.

Another interesting thing is that in the wild, horses naturally maintain the condition of their teeth by chewing on rocks to file down sharp edges that could interfere with their ability to chew correctly. Their jaw is also designed to move in a circular motion, helping the teeth to grind the forage and begin the process of digestion. Routine dental care to keep nature's system working is important. Healthy teeth and jaws are vital for proper digestion of the stalled horse's food. Working with these natural design considerations will go a long way toward not only helping your horse's digestive system, but also making him or her more comfortable.

Nutritional Things to Keep In Mind

Regular feed times – horses are creatures of habit and they have a built-in body clock that lets them know when it's feeding time. Delaying or missing a feeding can not only have a physical effect in terms of upsetting energy levels, but can also have a psychological effect, causing worry, stress and related behavioral issues. More frequent feedings at smaller but regular intervals will aid the natural digestive system of the horse, promoting safer absorption and reducing the anxiety levels of most horses. I'm not stating here that irregular feeding will necessarily destroy your horse, but it's my opinion that they are just more relaxed if they know when to expect their food.

Allow time for digestion before riding – try to allow an hour after feeding before starting your session, particularly after a large feeding or when a hard riding session is planned. You only need to consider how you yourself would feel if attempting to exercise on a full stomach to appreciate how uncomfortable your horse would feel, and how it might affect their willingness or behavior.

Water before a feeding – horses need to drink often. It's essential that *clean* water is *always* available. A lack of water will reduce feed intake and can cause dehydration, which will affect the overall function of the digestive system. A lack of water also increases the risk of impaction colic, which can have serious consequences. If a water bucket has been emptied or knocked over, or an automatic system is dirty or contaminated in any way, a horse will usually not drink enough. Water should be provided before offering feed. The "little and often" principal of intake is of vital importance to avoid the potential for guzzling large amounts and overfilling the stomach.

Feed Basics

- **Forage**

  Bulky hay or grasses are what we commonly call "long-stem forage." Pastures provide the most natural forage for horses. Domestic pastures need to be examined, analyzed and rotated, and have constant manure control to be able to offer proper nutrition for a horse. Stalled horses are quite opposite to pastured horses that graze throughout the day. Their nutritional needs require a much closer look. Many varieties of hay are available for the stalled or partially pastured horse. It would be too difficult to cover all of them in this chapter. The most important thing to note is that when in good general health, horses need an appropriate amount of good quality hay, at regular intervals, on a daily basis. Long-stem forage enhances digestion for horses, much as fiber does for humans. Because it takes time to chew, it helps prevent undesirable boredom-related behavior, such as wood chewing or tail chewing etc.

Soils are being depleted and over-used these days, which can't help but deplete the nutrients in the hay that is available to our horses. I recommend that you ask a reputable feed dealer to give you a short course on the hay choices available in your area. If possible, get an explanation of the benefits of each and then have your hay of choice analyzed for content. This will help to familiarize you with the nutrients: protein, fat, fiber, ash and mineral content of the hay you're feeding your horse. Again, forage is the mainstay of the typical horse's diet and should, in most cases, be the largest portion of their daily feeding. Lack of good forage, or forage filled with dust, mold, weeds, foreign material, rodent fecal matter or insect infestation can lead to many irreversible health problems or toxicity. *Note that any change in diet should be done gradually over a period of several days to allow the digestive tract to adapt to any new feed.*

- **Complete Feeds**

Today's brands of "complete feeds" are formulated to provide your horse with everything he or she needs. However, unless you have a horse that can't chew or digest long-stem forage, the reality is that complete feeds deprive a horse of the roughage they need to keep their gut moving. The forage content of manufactured complete feed is too fine to aid digestion in the same way that grass or hay does. Complete feeds *can* be used in limited amounts to round out and supplement a balanced diet, much as a multi-vitamin does for a human.

- **Sweet Feeds**

Any feedstuff that contains added sugar, usually in the form of molasses, is a 'sweet feed.' This category, contrary to popular belief, includes both loose grain feeds *and* feeds that come in pellet form. You may not be able to see the molasses in a pellet, but by taking the time to read and understand the tag on the bag, you will discover how much sugar it actually contains. Many folks base their decision to feed sweet feeds purely on cost. However, manufacturers might only be able to keep pricing low by using low cost ingredients. Even expensive, quality sweet feeds may still contain high amounts of sugar. The sugar highs and lows and associated behavioral issues seen in children subjected to a diet of sugar can also be seen in horses that are getting sugar added to their diet. Not only is excess sugar bad for human consumption, it's bad for our horses too.

Reading Feed Tags

The ingredients listed on a feed tag can be long and intimidating, but the most important thing to realize is that the ingredients are listed in weight order, so the ingredient at the top of the list makes up the highest proportion of the product. Ideally, the first few items on the list should be a form of forage, such as mixed hay or alfalfa meal, as these will provide your horse with the fiber needed to aid digestion. However, if the main ingredients are grains, it's important to know that sugar and starch contents will vary depending on the source. Corn, for example, has higher sugar content than oats.

Many of the lower cost feeds list the main ingredient as "grain products" without stating exactly which grains are included. This makes it hard to know if the content is appropriate for your horse's nutritional needs *and* temperament. It also makes it impossible to know whether the grain content of each new bag you open matches the content of the last bag. The grain content may vary from week to week depending on which one is most readily available to the manufacturer and for what price. I recommend that you only buy brands that clearly list the individual ingredients, so that you know what you're actually giving your horse.

What Is in Your Horse's Diet?

If your veterinarian asked you to provide the exact details of your horse's daily diet, could you? Could you quote the weight of forage given daily? Do you know your horse's weight, and if so, what percentage of his weight you're giving in feed? How much of that is forage and how much falls into the other categories? If you feed your horse one of the many popular complete feeds, sweet feeds, or feeds that come in pellet form, do you know *exactly* what's in the bag? Most folks know how many flakes, or what they think is a flake, their horses are getting, but don't know the actual weight of the flake. Weight is more important than the number of flakes, as an average flake of grass hay can vary anywhere from two to five pounds, or more. An average flake of alfalfa can weigh up to eight pounds or more. Knowing at least basic nutritional information is vital to caring for your horse's health.

Choosing the Right Feed for Your Horse

Many horse owners choose a brand or type of feed purely on the recommendations of someone else, maybe be a store clerk or stable mate. Horse owners might buy whatever others are using, or what might be available at their boarding facility. I've personally seen very nice barns feed terrible hay. If you value your horse's nutrition, be sure to examine the hay supply when touring a new facility as carefully as you do the wash racks, etc.

The right feed for your horse must not only provide the energy needed to perform, but it also must suit *them*. Unfortunately, when a horse becomes "high" or excitable on the feed they're being given, many people choose to just feed less. They don't consider the need to try a *different type* of feed. Limiting the ration may only result in the horse becoming malnourished from inadequate intake of essential nutrients and forage weight.

Of course, feeding *more* than the recommended ration, mixing complete feeds, or adding extra ingredients to scientifically formulated feedstuffs can also create an imbalance. This highlights the importance of understanding *exactly* what's in your horse's diet. Gaining that understanding means paying attention to the total amount of food consumed, including the quality, the amount of grazing they have access to, and taking the time to read the feed tags on the bags you use.

Feeding Guidelines

As a general rule of thumb, a horse in a moderate exercise program needs the equivalent of 1.5 to 2 percent of his or her bodyweight in food per day to maintain weight, including both forage and grains. In the wild, this would consist of forage only, and again would be consumed on a "little and often" basis through continual grazing. For this reason, giving three or four small feedings spread across the day is preferable to only two larger feedings. It's recommended that at least 1 percent of the 1.5% to 2% weight in food should be long-stem forage. In the case of a stalled horse's diet, the long-stemmed fiber content of hay is preferable to the short-stemmed fiber provided by a complete feed. When appropriate, hay given on an ad-lib basis can also alleviate boredom and limit the potential for a horse to bolt, or wolf down, his or her feed when it appears.

> **BEFORE THE CROP COMES OUT…KEY POINT TO CONSIDER NUMBER 5**
>
> **A MALNOURISHED HORSE SIMPLY CAN'T GIVE YOU THEIR PHYSICAL OR MENTAL BEST.**

What is the Right Amount of Food?

This depends on two things: your horse's weight, and their level of activity. Before you can figure out how much food your horse needs, you must first figure out how much he or she weighs. Gaining access to weighing scales suitable for a large animal isn't always an option, so a simpler solution is to use a weight tape. This tape can help approximate a horse's weight.

Measuring Your Horse's Weight with a Tape

Weight tapes are soft measuring tapes calibrated in pounds instead of inches. They're available from most tack or feed stores. It takes practice to obtain a reasonably accurate reading, so each measurement should be taken three times and the average used as the final figure.

- Make sure your horse is standing squarely on a flat surface. (Fig. 5.1)
- Make sure he or she is relaxed. This is particularly important in relation to head position as it can lead to big differences in measurements. (Fig. 5.2)
- Standing on your horse's left, holding the zero end of the tape in your hand, position the remaining tape over his or her back so that it hangs down on the right side of their body in the same way and place that a girth or cinch would. (Fig. 5.3)
- Keeping hold of the zero end, reach under your horse to bring the rest of the tape around under their heart girth. This is an indentation where the cinch would naturally find its home. Form a complete loop around the body. (Fig. 5.4)
- Pull the tape gently in order to get the most accurate reading. The number on the tape where it meets the zero end is your horse's weight (make sure the tape is not twisted). (Fig. 5.5)

In order to assess if your horse needs more or less food currently, the Horse Body Condition Scoring is a guide that can be used (based on a system devised by C.L. Carroll and P.J. Huntington: "Body Condition Scoring and Weight Estimation of Horses," *Equine Veterinary Journal* 20, 21-45, 1988). If you have health concerns over your horse's weight, you can always seek expert advice from your veterinarian.

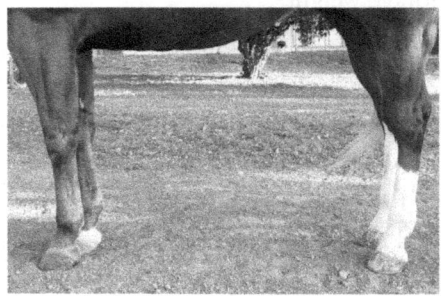

Figure 5.1 Square the horse up on a flat surface.

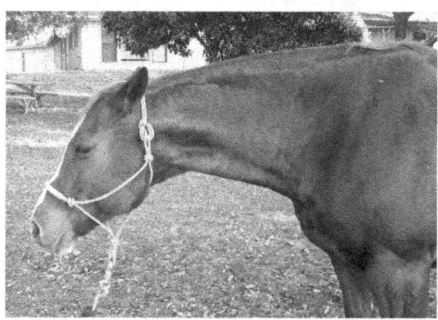

Figure 5.2 Make sure the horse's head is relaxed as a raised head can give a different measurement.

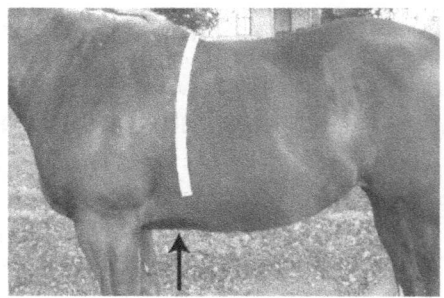

Figure 5.3 Position the tape near the withers in perpendicular alignment with the heart girth. The heart girth is the indentation where the cinch would naturally gravitate towards. The natural home of the cinch.

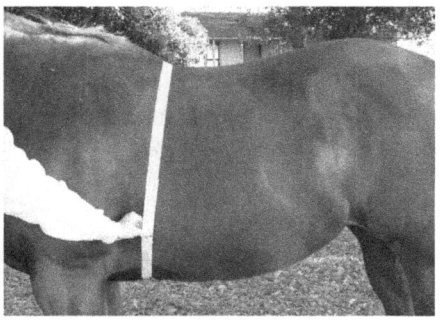
Figure 5.4 Bring the tape around to a snug fit to read the weight measurement.

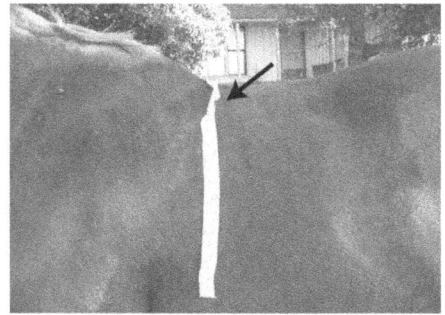
Figure 5.5 Be sure that you do not twist the tape.

Horse Body Condition Scoring

This method uses a scale of 1 to 9 with 1 representing extremely thin and 9 representing obese. A horse is considered to be at an ideal weight when they score around the middle of the scale. Scoring is determined by comparing your horse's appearance and the feel of their body against listed criteria. It's beyond the scope of this chapter to list every detail of the scoring system but the main points are outlined below.

SCORE	CONDITION	APPEARANCE
1	Emaciated	The bony structures of the hips, ribs, shoulders and withers are clearly visible and the spinous processes are prominent. No fatty tissue can be felt.
2	Very thin	As above, with bony structures only slightly less prominent than in an emaciated horse.

NUTRITION AND DENTAL 57

SCORE	CONDITION	APPEARANCE
3	Thin	A slight covering of fat over the ribs. Neck and shoulders less noticeably thin, but bony structures still visible.
4	Moderately thin	Hips less prominent with a slight layer of fat along the top line and over the hindquarters.
5	Moderate	Neck, withers, shoulders and buttocks have a more rounded appearance. The ribs are no longer visible but can be felt easily by hand.
6	Moderately fleshy	A more rounded appearance as above with the ribs no longer felt easily.

SCORE	CONDITION	APPEARANCE
7	Fleshy	Fat deposits can be felt on the neck, withers and shoulders. A slight crease (dip) appears in the flesh along the length of the back.
8	Fat	As above, with noticeably more thickening of the neck and the wither area, and clearly visible fat deposits on the buttocks.
9	Extremely fat	As above, with visible fat deposits also noticeable on the ribs, creating a bulging appearance on the neck and over the shoulders and withers.

Feed Rations and Your Horse's Level of Activity

The correct amount of food to give your horse can only be measured by first knowing their weight and then by understanding his or her level of activity. It's extremely important *not* to overestimate the amount of exercise your horse actually does. Exercise is commonly categorized as being light, moderate, or heavy, but many owners or riders are unable or unwilling to recognize the category that best fits their horse's level of activity.

*Overestimating the level of activity leads to overfeeding.
An overfed horse is an unhealthy, and often unhappy horse.*

Basic exercise levels:

- **Light exercise** = up to three hours per week of recreational riding or conditioning, mainly walk and trot with limited periods of cantering.
- **Moderate exercise** = up to five hours per week of recreational riding, including faster paced work and technical skills such as jumping, showing, or ranch work.
- **Heavy exercise** = four or five hours per week of strenuous effort including faster paced work, skills training, regular and frequent showing, ranch work, jumping events, or preparation for lower level racing.

*Only by being realistic about your horse's weight and amount of
exercise can you provide them with the correct amount
of food to meet their nutritional needs.*

Weight Management

The key to successfully achieving and maintaining your horse's optimum weight is to measure it regularly, adjust food intake for the amount of exercise, and monitor the results. If your horse is gaining or losing weight beyond the ideal range, you must make the necessary adjustments to their dietary intake to regain balance. To reduce body fat, reduce the amount of feed by 25 percent. If your horse is too thin, just reverse this process and add 25 percent more food. After attaining the ideal weight, increase or decrease the amount of feed slowly and play with rations until you're satisfied that your horse is maintaining the desired weight. If something seems wrong, adjust accordingly.

Malnutrition and Sugar Behavioral Issues

There is growing evidence that many equine behavioral issues are the result of malnutrition. These issues may be remedied or avoided if you pay close attention to your horse's individual diet. It's also widely recognized that certain foods can trigger allergic or behavioral reactions—the adverse effects of high sugar content is a good example. Horses are just as susceptible to sugars in their diet and weight related health problems as humans are.

*A malnourished horse is very often an over 'emotional' horse,
prone to being excitable, irritable, unable to focus, or overreacting
in new or stressful situations.*

Routine Dental Care – A Must!

Choosing the right feedstuff for your horse and feeding the correct quantity of food are important elements of providing your horse with adequate nutrition. However, even the most carefully considered and balanced diet will fall short of providing your horse with the nutrition they need if they're unable to chew and digest it properly.

Common signs of dental issues are:
- Loss of condition
- Inability to chew efficiently
- Large particles of grain in droppings
- Bolting (gulping) feed
- Dunking hay in water
- Excessive dribbling or dropping of food when eating
- Bad breath
- Inability to collect (locked TMJ).

Dental issues will not only have a direct impact on your horse's ability to eat and gain maximum nutrition from their daily ration of food, they can also affect his or her behavior or lead to impaction colic. These will most likely manifest as symptoms such as:

- Irregular movement of the lower jaw
- Head shaking when ridden
- Rearing or bucking when ridden
- Pulling against the bit and rider
- Avoiding the bit and not accepting the bit
- Sores or soft tissue injuries on the inside of the mouth
- Poor attitude and general head shyness.

Horses should have their teeth "floated" or at least checked once a year. Floating is a process where a file or tool is used to smooth or contour a horse's teeth, which unlike human teeth, keep growing; they develop points or sharp edges over time, making it hard or uncomfortable to chew or hold a bit. It's good to remember that many of the above symptoms can also be connected to an inappropriate bit choice—discussed in Chapter 4—just doing your best to provide your horse with balanced nutrition and optimum dental care will go a long way.

Grace's Dental Story

Grace had her annual float or dental work done each year. During a routine visit from a new equine dentist, it was discovered that her jaw was locked at the temporomandibular joint, also known as the TMJ. This locked jaw wouldn't allow her to pull the lower teeth back in her head as a horse needs to do in order to collect correctly. You can demonstrate this on yourself. Tuck your chin to your chest and feel the sensation of your lower jaw pulling backward as you do so. If your jaw were locked in place, you would feel tension every time you put your head down. This is what Grace was experiencing when asked to collect. This is just another small thing that might be overlooked, that can make a big difference to our animals, I know that it has with my own horse. Grace is much more compliant now that this has been corrected.

CHAPTER 6

Conditioning and Stretching

Grace's Story

Grace had been bought for the 'grandkids' to ride. After the kids lost interest, now given to ATVs and motorcycles, she stood in a pasture eating all day. When I bought her, she hadn't been ridden for quite some time. I was lucky in that when I did choose a trainer, I met someone who understood the horse as an athlete. After two years of learning and studying with someone with that athletic thought process, I had a good understanding of how to approach conditioning, along with many other aspects of the horse from a physiological basis. Again, horses and humans are not that different. My own personal experience of going to the gym and of personal fitness training helped me to understand the importance of warm ups, stretches, aerobic and muscle strength training programs, and days of rest. These are exactly the same needs for the horse, as athlete. I'm sincerely thankful that I met a person with such a unique physical understanding of the horse in the early stages of my own learning.

It's not uncommon for me to see a rider get on their horse and go straight into loping around the arena within just a few minutes. It seems that the fast-paced way of life many of us now lead keeps us in a constant state of rushing. We expect our horses to be able to spring straight into action from the moment we tack up and hop on. No matter how intense the workload is about to become on the horse's body during the ride ahead, a round or two of walking seems to be considered adequate preparation time for most riders. Sadly, when this is the case, both horse *and* rider are missing out on an essential element of any exercise routine: the warm up.

The Warm Up

Warm up – a period or act of preparation for a game, performance, or exercise session, involving gentle exercise or practice. This warm up for horses can take up to 20 minutes.

If you've ever been involved in any kind of sports activity, taken part in exercise classes or attended a gym, you will most likely be aware of the emphasis placed on warming up. Your muscles need to warm up appropriately for the activity ahead and for the challenges your body will face. Warm muscles are more flexible, so they're better able to perform in terms of providing strength, speed, endurance or any other physical movement required in your chosen activity; they're also less susceptible to injury when performing those movements. Top professional athletes often have very complex, lengthy warm up routines designed to progressively prepare every inch of their bodies for the intense efforts of producing a world-class performance, but warming up is not just for Olympians.

Horses by nature are designed to be constantly on the move. This continual movement aids in the circulation of blood, keeps the muscles warm, promotes flexibility and maintains the range of movement around the joints, all of which is nature's way of keeping a horse in a constant state of readiness should they need to flee from danger.

All *horses and* all *riders, at* all *levels benefit equally from being appropriately prepared for* every *exercise session.*

Getting your horse on the move by walking him or her in-hand before riding is a good way to begin the warm up process, especially if they're normally confined to the restricted space of a stall for the majority of the day. When available, a hot walker can provide a convenient alternative to walking in-hand, but time must be taken to train your horse in its use so that it can be used safely. A good warm up is essential to a good ride. It can take a horse up to 20 minutes to suitably warm up. This is a benchmark for a good start to a ride.

Simple Stretches (figs. 6.1 - 6.4)

Simple stretches are an integral part of any warm up routine for your own body. Once your muscles become warmer and more flexible, simple stretches continue to prepare your body for the activity ahead by gradually increasing the range of movement around your joints. This same principle should be applied to your horse's body with

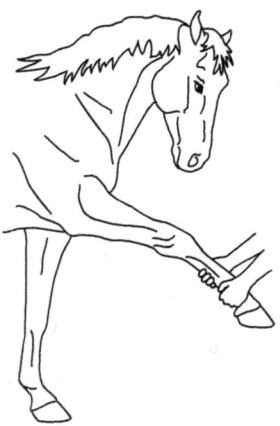

Figure 6.1 Front leg stretch.

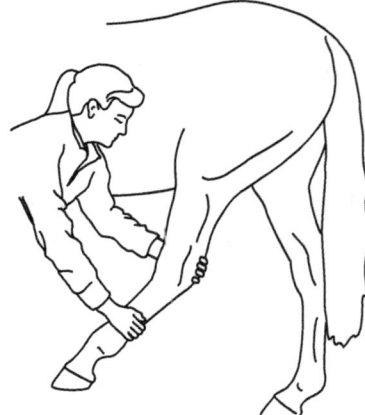

Figure 6.2 Hind leg stretch.

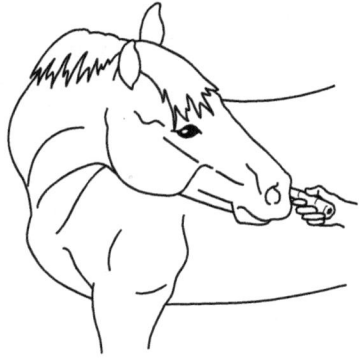 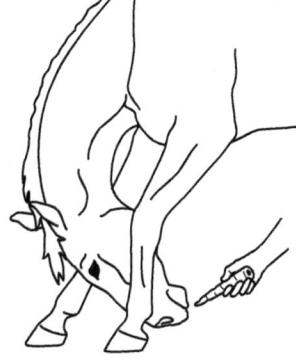

Figure 6.3 Carrot stretch to the side.   **Figure 6.4** Carrot stretch down and between.

the idea being that simple, low intensity movements via simple stretches can begin to gradually increase the flexibility of the working muscles without overstretching them. Simple stretching is best done after a period of time on the hot walker or after a bit of hand walking, as the preliminary warm up affords the muscles their best stretch. Although there are only a few examples pictured here, there are several resources available that feature a more elaborate assortment of stretches. The *Masterson Method*™ techniques mentioned in chapter 2 are also a good precursor to exercise.

> **BEFORE THE CROP COMES OUT…KEY POINT TO CONSIDER NUMBER 6**
>
> **POOR BEHAVIOR COULD BE THE RESULT OF POOR CONDITIONING.**

Preparing and Judging the Correct Amount of Exercise

Another essential element of conditioning is ensuring that your horse receives the correct amount of exercise to keep him or her fit for their intended purpose. A racehorse in training requires an entirely different conditioning program than a horse being ridden purely for pleasure, but in both cases, the amount of conditioning and the intensity of the program must be appropriate to the level of fitness required.

If your goal is to increase your horse's level of fitness, you must have an accurate understanding exactly how fit or unfit they are now. This means being aware of the amount of exercise your horse is currently doing and paying attention to the intensity. For example, if you are a runner or a swimmer, you probably know exactly what distance you're able to cover within a set period of time. You will also be aware of what pace you're able to maintain over that period.

To achieve any goal, you need clear steps to help you get there.

With this in mind, you should make yourself aware of your horse's cardio and endurance capabilities, how much time they spend in a certain gait, how long they can maintain it, etc. For example, if your goal is a reining pattern, or a round of jumping, your horse needs to be conditioned to perform for at least that required length of time. Can your horse trot for 15 minutes straight? Can they lope or canter for 10 or 20 minutes? Don't just guess how long the routine is. Use a clock and time your rides, then take note at what point your horse begins to fatigue. After assessing that, you can set yourself a series of smaller targets to help you progress towards a more ambitious goal. If you want to increase fitness and improve condition, increase the amount of exercise gradually in small increments, such as a minute or two each ride, until the desired length of time is achieved. Always divide your time going both directions for balance.

If you're working on conditioning, don't just drift around aimlessly, ride with a purpose. After all, improving your horse's fitness and achieving peak condition isn't just about spending time in the saddle. It's not the amount of time you put into each session that counts, it's what you put into that time that matters.

The Boredom Factor

Even when in top condition, a horse may still show reluctance, or under-perform when ridden. They may be simply bored or by their routine. If you slip into a habit of always doing the same warm up routine or following the same pattern of movements each time you ride, your horse will simply switch off mentally and begin to operate on "automatic pilot", just as you would if forced to repeat the same actions over and over again. To maintain your horse's focus and enthusiasm, you must make sure that he or she is mentally as well as physically stimulated and engaged by keeping variety in their routine. Cross training is something we seem to have lost sight of, or as horse owners, have never thought about in the first place. Studies have shown that human athletes benefit from cross training in preparation for high caliber athletic performances. Our horses do, too. For example, if you're a Dressage rider and you only do the same drills in the arena, over and over, you may find that your horse is just going through the motions to "get through" the session. Some horses even memorize the patterns. Many of our animals are stoic and compliant to a fault, but if you take that same Dressage horse and do a bit of jumping, obstacles or trail riding through the hills for building strength, just feel the difference in concentration you get the next time you get into the arena.

Be Fair

We always want to set our horses up to succeed, so we need to set tasks that they can achieve. For example, if you're jumping, make sure you build slowly to the height, width and speed of an individual jump or course. Be careful not to "over-face" the horse (ask too much, too soon). Be considerate and thoughtful. Starting a baby off by jumping a three-foot fence isn't fair, no matter how excited you are to see him or her go over it.

Don't forget the Cool Down

Understanding the need to cool down properly is important, as lactic acid, produced in the muscle tissue during strenuous exercise, will build and remain pent up inside the muscle belly and attachments unless it is allowed to release through a cooling off period. To properly cool off, be sure to walk the horse until the muscles are cool to the touch and breathing has regulated back to normal.

Preventing Injury

Be flexible in your approach to conditioning, and in tune with your horse's immediate needs. Impatience to reach a goal—set by the rider—can end up resulting in conflict or even worse, injury. It's my belief that because horses read intentions and are so sensitive, rushing through our routine with our horses could become a source of stress, resentment or disappointment, both for us and for our horses. These attitudes can permeate our own physical state and translate down into our horse's bodies, thus creating the same physical sensations in them. A horse working under stress can be an injury waiting to happen, and this can compound if left unchecked over time.

We have to be mindful of just how connected our horses can actually be with our intentions.

We've all had days where, even with the best of intentions, we've set goals for ourselves but failed to achieve them. Changes in weather conditions, for example, may cause you to change your schedule. Other factors such as tiredness or tight muscles may also create the need to make a change of plan. Just as the efforts of your last treadmill session in the gym, or a close and desperate game of outdoor soccer may have left your own muscles feeling fatigued for a number of days, there's a very good chance that your horse may have experienced the same fatigue symptoms after your last ride or session. The challenge is that he or she can't tell you so. On the other hand, your horse might also have increased energy on a particular day and that energy may not line up with the precise and detailed program you had planned, such as side passing, turns on the haunches, or a difficult Dressage move. Without the ability and flexibility to bend your program to your horse's needs, you might find yourself in an unnecessary fight. By learning to read in your horse what you have *coming out* of the stall each day, you learn to assess the best program ahead for both of you. There's nothing wrong with adapting your plans, after all, that's what we expect our horses to do. Knowing when it's appropriate to ask for more from your horse and when to ease back is an intuitive skill that can only be mastered through taking the time to really *know* your horse. You are, in fact, your horse's 'personal trainer'. The hard truth is, if your impatience for progress leads to mistaking soreness for "laziness," or pushing your horse to do more before they're able to recover from the last hard workout, the result may be the beginnings of an injury, or worse. The damage done may halt your progress indefinitely.

The Weekend Trail Ride

Fit for a purpose applies to *all* purposes, even when your sole purpose is to ride purely for pleasure. All too often, pleasure riders keep their horses confined in unnaturally small stalls for days or weeks at a time, then suddenly on a weekend afternoon decide to take their horse out on a four-hour trail ride through the hills. You only have to imagine how your own body would feel if subjected to the same treatment after weeks of sitting around on your couch to understand why being aware of your horse's condition and welfare is important. Just because they're large animals doesn't mean they can take whatever we dish out, nor should they be expected to do so whenever it suits *our* whim. Fitness can't be stored, so getting your horse into condition and then maintaining that condition requires a progressive training program of *regular* exercise. It's an unfortunate fact that a great many injuries in horses are the result of the rider failing to understand the importance of matching their horse's fitness and condition to the amount of exercise they expect them to do. A four-hour trail ride can only be a pleasure ride if both you *and* your horse are in suitable condition to remain comfortable for the duration.

The Equine Athlete

Human athletes are very much in tune with their bodies and are extremely aware of aches, pains or minute amounts of muscle tightness that could potentially be a sign of trouble if left untreated. In short, they know how to *listen* to their body. They understand their bodies and can gauge for themselves whether they just need to give their muscles a little more time to warm up, take it a little easier than planned in the workout session ahead, or take a complete rest. Your horse is an equine athlete who is just as susceptible to those same aches, pains and tightness in their muscles as you are, but again, he or she can't tell you in words how they're feeling. However, they can tell you in other ways. Your horse *will show you* if you take the time to look at them in a new light, have the desire to read their body and facial language, and learn how to *listen* to what your horse is telling you through their actions.

By being able to detect our horse's physical issues, we can correct or eliminate many sources of conflict or unwanted behavior that otherwise baffle or frustrate us. It's times like these when we presume the horse is at fault, and we try all the harder to control them. Confused by his or her need to communicate with you, trying to communicate, yet being disciplined for communicating, your horse slips into a downward cycle, slowly dying inside.

CHAPTER 7

Grooming and Husbandry

Our Story

I have always loved grooming. It became apparent to me that I was always the first to start and the last to finish when it came to getting Grace ready to ride. After so many comments about her shining coat from others, and about how much they would love their own horses to have such a coat, I realized that my thorough grooming both before and after a ride was contributing not only to our time together, but also to her amazing coat. It was only after a long time caring for Grace that I began to observe how grooming actually contributed to our relationship.

Grooming is so much more than a cleaning process; it's an opportunity to get to know your horse for that day. People who rush through it might see it as something that eats into their riding time, but grooming is actually a valuable bonding process that has the potential to enhance, not take away from their ride that day. In fact, grooming sets the tone for everything. If you're working at a hurried pace and feeling pressed for time, your horse will pick up on it and more likely than not, mirror the same attitude. The same can be said of your mood, if you begin the grooming process feeling anxious or in a bad mood about the events of the day, that mood is conveyed to your horse. Don't forget: horses read your intentions.

The way you groom sets the tone for the ride or session ahead.

The way you approach grooming or handling not only sets the tone for the ride ahead, it also has the potential to affect the entire relationship. If you expect your horse to give you his or her best, you must give them your best by taking the time to work around them with love, care, consideration and RESPECT.

Reasons for Grooming

The most obvious reason for grooming is general cleanliness, but it also adds to the bonding experience between you and your horse. Thorough grooming involves paying attention to your horse's entire body. When you get into the habit of brushing your horse from head to toe, top to bottom, you get to know every square inch of them. This allows you to pick up on tiny changes that could lead to serious or significant problems

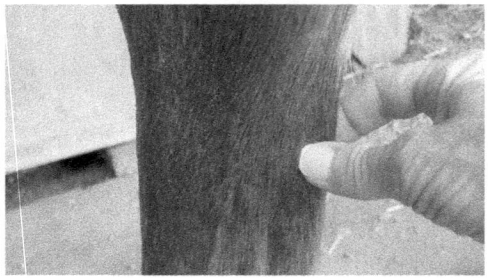

Figure 7.1 Checking tendons should be done with a very light or feather like touch.

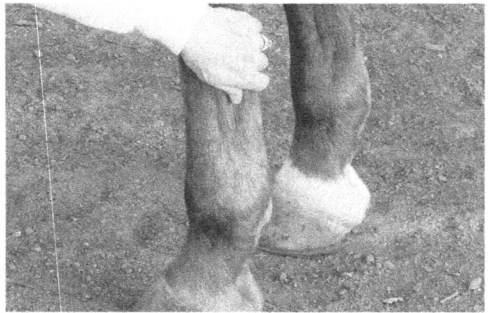

Figure 7.2 Check tendons daily.

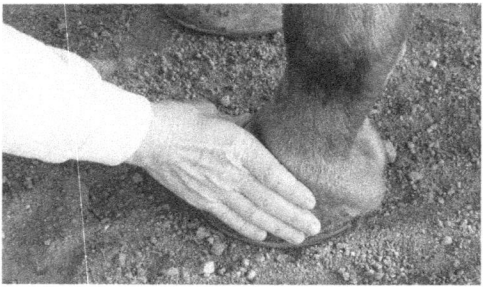

Figure 7.3 Check hooves daily.

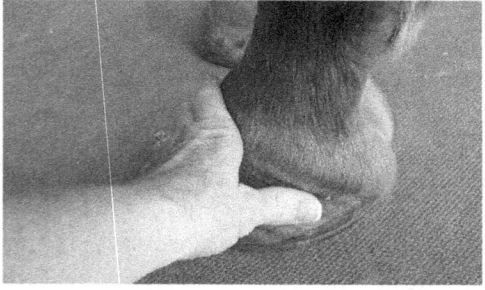

Figure 7.4 Founder can sometimes be avoided or minimized if caught early enough.

that might otherwise go unnoticed. It makes it possible to notice things such as embedded ticks, swellings, scratches, wounds, tight muscles or inflamed tendons. Of course, not every lump or bump on your horse's body is necessarily a sign of a major problem, but you have to know what "normal" is for your horse before you can spot changes that might indicate that things are not as they should be. If you hurry through grooming, you might miss things that could potentially lead to bigger problems. For example, a dirty tail might indicate dietary or digestive problems; an itchy mane might indicate a skin irritation or parasite problem. Heat or swelling usually indicates injury, infection or a disruption of normal tissue.

It's particularly important to check these areas daily: legs, feet, and hocks. Leg tendons should be felt with a feather-light touch down the back of each tendon (Fig. 7.1). This light touch allows you to feel small changes from normal texture, temperature or swelling (Fig. 7.2).

Knowing the normal temperature of your horse's feet, both before and after exercise (Fig. 7.3), might help you detect a developing issue. Anything other than normal can indicate a challenge with the hoof system. For example, the early detection of heat or a pulse in the hoof as in a case of founder (also known as laminitis – a rotation or sinking of the coffin bone in the hoof caused by inflammation) might actually save your horse's life (Fig. 7.4).

Hocks (Fig. 7.5) and knees should also be checked regularly for heat and swelling. These are also complicated areas of anatomy where horses can develop troubles long before lameness shows.

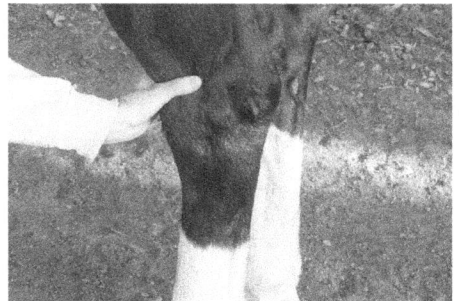

Figure 7.5 Check hocks daily.

Your horse can't tell you how they feel, but they can show you in other ways. By paying attention to every detail of your horse's body, you might pick up on important indicators of potential pain or discomfort that could be affecting his or her behavior.

Grooming Essentials

When it comes to choosing items for your grooming box, there seems to be no end to the number of products available. What matters most is how they work for you and how they make your horse feel.

My grooming box contains the following:

- Rubber curry comb.
- Stiff body brush.
- Hand mitt with a "knobby" texture.
- Two medium body brushes (hand size).
- Soft body brush or finishing brush.
- Mane and tail brush.
- Hoof pick with brush.
- Household or all-purpose cloths.
- Wound medication and soothing cream for sores or wounds.
- Fly spray during fly season (also fly wipe for the face).
- Dry thrush product for the treatment of thrush (see recommended resources).
- Braiding bands for tying up the forelock and tail and a stitch remover for cutting out braids.
- *Farnam™ Excalibur* sheath cleaner, a product designed to soften and ease the cleaning process of the "crud" in delicate areas and can also be used on the front cannon bone area of the rear legs.

Intuitive grooming lets you assess your horse's mood.

The more time you spend grooming, the more you get to know your horse and the more intuitive the process becomes. When you are able to recognize your horse's moods as well as your own, you'll be able to change your ride or training plans accordingly. Disappointment and failure can be avoided so easily by simply taking the time to understand your horse's mood *before* you hop on their back.

A Grooming Routine

Just as you might have developed your own personal grooming habits and routines, you will also develop your own preferred method of grooming your horse. The order in which you do things isn't important. What *is* important is that you do it properly. With this in mind, the more routine your thorough grooming procedure becomes, the more skilled you will become in terms of noticing any tiny changes, making it less likely that you will miss something small but ultimately significant.

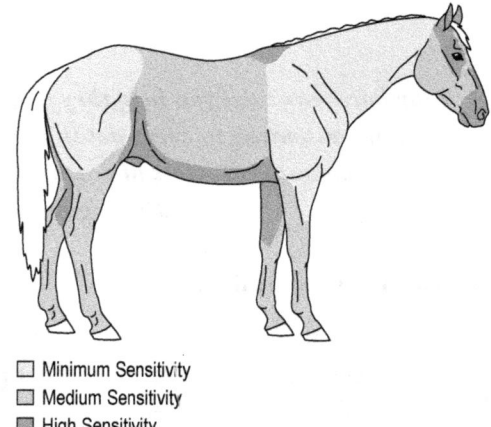

☐ Minimum Sensitivity
☐ Medium Sensitivity
■ High Sensitivity

Figure 7.6 Sensitivity chart for grooming

The *whys* for each brush:

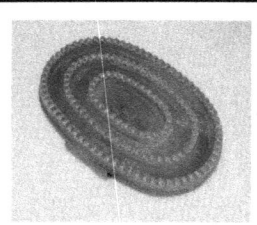	**Rubber curry comb** – the flexibility of a rubber curry, when used in a circular motion, provides a massaging effect which stimulates the blood flow and aids circulation. It should be used with care on the sensitive areas of the body (Fig. 7.6).
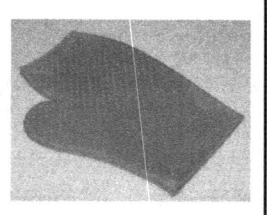	**"Knobby" hand mitt** – the raised rubber pimples on a grooming mitt are ideal for loosening surface dirt and hair on the more sensitive bony areas such as the lower limbs and the face. My own mare particularly enjoys the sensation of the mitt around her face, on her forehead and under her jaw in the throat latch area. Her enjoyment allows me to thoroughly groom those potentially awkward areas and, just as importantly, allows her to start her day in a positive, calm and relaxed mood.

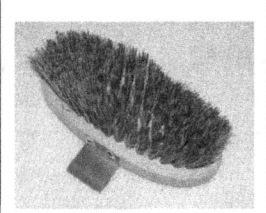	**Stiff body brush** – the purpose of this brush is to remove the dirt and hair already loosened by the use of the rubber curry comb. This brush is not suitable for use in sensitive areas.
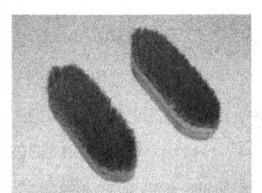	**Medium body brushes** – I use two small hand held medium bristle brushes to work out more dirt and hair after the stiff brush. These brushes can be used in some of the more sensitive areas as well. I like small brushes that fit my small hands, as I seem to be able to hold on to them better. I can also use two at a time, one on each side of the legs simultaneously. One of these brushes can be used as a good start to the face after the knobby mitt has loosened hair and dirt.
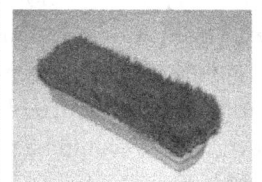	**Soft body and face brush** – also known as a finishing brush, the bristles on a soft brush are generally longer than those on a stiff or medium brush as well as much finer and denser. The soft bristles penetrate deeper into the coat to remove the remaining dust and hair, creating a finished appearance and shine. For this reason, a soft brush is best used in conjunction with a metal curry comb. The metal curry comb was designed to remove the dirt from a brush, cleaning it while you work. *It's important to note that a metal curry comb is for brushes only* and was *never* designed to be used on your horse's body. Also, your soft brush can be used to groom the sensitive areas of the head and face along with the lower legs. I always take the time to cup my hand over my horse's eye and protect it from dust or hair going straight into the eye.
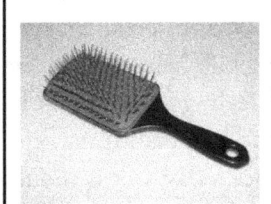	**Mane and tail brush** – the purpose of a mane and tail brush is to detangle the hairs without causing excessive breakage or pulling too many of them out. Any human hair brush that you would enjoy brushing your own long hair with is suitable for this purpose. Take the time to carefully brush out the tangles from the bottom first and work your way up toward the roots on both the mane and tail. This method causes the least amount of breakage and discomfort. 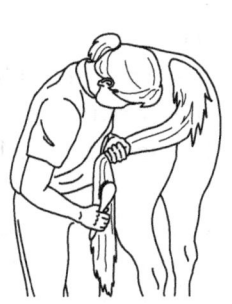

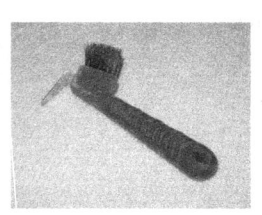	**Hoof pick** – along with removing dirt, feces, urine and potentially harmful stones, picking out the hooves provides an opportunity to check the overall condition of each hoof and to check for thrush or any other variation from the norm. The importance of maintaining healthy hooves is detailed in chapter 1. For best results, it's always good to pick hooves both before and after a ride.
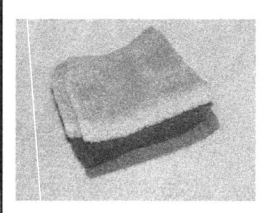	**Eyes, nostrils and ears** – using a clean damp cloth to wipe eye areas, nostrils and ears provides an opportunity to check for and remove any debris, unusual discharges or other foreign objects as well as leaving your horse feeling fresh and ready for the ride ahead. This also helps keep flies out of the eye area which can clog tear ducts, giving your horse that weepy eye look and worse yet, a potential vet bill to clear the ducts.

The above grooming routine can take up to a half hour to complete. I personally groom both before and after each ride. I also clean delicate areas almost daily. These areas are different on mares than on geldings or stallions. Each will require a different technique. The only way to make it a less "delicate" procedure is to get your horse accustomed to you working in those private areas. Shying away from it or skipping over it is of no benefit to your horse in the long run. Take the time to clean these areas carefully and with respect. If needed, work with a professional until you're comfortable with this on your own. You only have to imagine how uncomfortable you would be to appreciate how important it is to look after your horse's personal hygiene.

Good animal husbandry requires a respectful approach.

Horse Husbandry Considerations

- **Stall Cleanliness**

    It stands to reason that the more comfortable your horse is in his or her environment, the happier they're going to be. If your horse is unable to relax because they don't have enough bedding or are being plagued by flies because of dirty bedding, they simply can't be expected to be relaxed. A thorough grooming will help set the tone for the ride ahead, but if your horse has already spent the day feeling uncomfortable, he or she may not be "in the mood" to perform the way you'd planned. It may not be possible to clean out your stall thoroughly more than once a day, but it should be routine practice to remove any visible droppings or urine each time you look in on your horse.

- **Hydration**

    Again, it's *essential* that your horse have an adequate supply of *fresh, clean water.*

- **Routine**

    Horses are creatures of habit. They thrive on routine and can quickly become upset when a routine is interrupted, especially if it has been established for a long time. This means that any changes to feeding times or any other daily routine must be made gradually. It also means that if the normal order of things in your horse's day has been disrupted in any way, the psychological effect may well manifest itself in your horse's behavior that day. This is of particular importance when going on the road. As one of my mentors once told me:

    "Going on the road can seem like your horse has 50 per cent less brain and 50 per cent more energy!"

    Maybe you've experienced this. Your horse simply can't be expected to instantly adapt to a new environment. Instinctively, they need to assess new situations for themselves; allowances must be made for behavior that's simply inbred in the horse. Take the time to show your horse around. You don't need to spend loads of time looking at each new object of your horse's concern at an event or new property. This can actually make things worse; just familiarize your horse with the new sights, smells and sounds that are going on in a broad but casual sense, without too much directed focus on your part. Focusing intently on something only makes it more important to your horse. After all, if you think it's worth looking at, your horse will follow your lead. This adjustment process will go a long way towards improving everyone's enjoyment of the day, especially if your horse doesn't get out to new places often. After you've developed a strong leadership position with your horse, or if that relationship has already evolved, your horse's ability to trust you in any new situation will become more and more evident to you. It will become less likely that you will have to go through the "introduction" procedure at new events or places. Once your horse trusts you completely, he or she will defer to your judgment on new things anywhere you go.

- **Organization**

    Organization is essential to every horse owner. To be able to provide the best care for your horse, you should maintain an accurate record of *everything* related to your horse's health and well being. For example, your horse needs to be kept on an appropriate worming program, shoeing must be checked and done at regular intervals, and vaccinations must be kept up to date. Try keeping a calendar at the ranch and marking it with appropriate dates and reminders. This can help you plan and remain organized. Without routine organization, it may be a behavioral issue instead of your calendar, which alerts you to the important "something" you've forgotten, or the treatment that is now overdue.

- **Keeping Your Horse at Home or Boarding Facility**

    Of course, there is much more to caring for your horse than grooming. Whether your horse is kept at a boarding stable or at home, they depend on you, or those whom you pay, to care and provide for them. Being in a position to keep your horse at home is often the ultimate dream of a horse owner, but it's important to remember that horses by nature are herd animals. You might find that they're actually happier in a boarding environment or at least with other horses, rather than in solitary confinement at your house. It's important to understand that even if you ride every day, your horse will spend the majority of his or her time alone. Without social interaction, a horse's boredom can lead to potential behavioral issues. The same principle can apply to horses in a boarding facility, but usually the close proximity to other horses and the general comings and goings of others helps to alleviate boredom. Access to paddocks and turnout areas will also provide a welcome distraction but again, natural instincts of the horse must be taken into consideration. Horses in the wild seek protection from danger by remaining with the herd. A horse turned out alone can become nervous or anxious about unfamiliar happenings, noises or smells. Even if your horse is turned out with other horses in the same pen, a natural pecking order will still develop among the group. The "fight" for dominance can result in injuries being inflicted or submissive animals being bullied and harassed. The point is that at the time of your ride, your horse's behavior is definitely going to be influenced by what has been going on in their day before you arrived. They may have become bored in their stall, anxious on their own, or withdrawn as a result of being bullied into a corner of the paddock by others. Their psychological state will have a direct impact on their physical behavior. These ideas might highlight the importance of intuitive grooming and understanding your horse's mood *before* you ride.

> **BEFORE THE CROP COMES OUT…KEY POINT TO CONSIDER NUMBER 7**
>
> **LOVE, CARE FOR, AND RESPECT YOUR HORSE TO BRING OUT THEIR BEST.**

Care with Respect

All aspects of grooming and horse husbandry should be approached as loving, caring components of horse ownership. Your motivation to provide the best care you can, must be driven by respect; a respect for your horse who so willingly gives you the best he or she can in return.

CHAPTER 8

Understanding Who You Are as a Rider and Choosing a Mentor

In wrapping up my thoughts on all of this, I began to evaluate the idea of teamwork. I was thinking about how much I appreciate the gift of my horse Grace and how blessed I am every day to be a partner for her. I'm amazed that I have such a wonderful creature to take care of in the first place. Through our challenges, we've learned *so* much together. I always have her best interests at heart, and hope to be the kind of owner every horse would want to have. That introspection has spawned this final chapter.

Who We Are as Riders

After exploring all the other possible things that might contribute to tension between you and your horse, there's one more question you must ask yourself: what commitment have you made to your horse? Horse ownership is really a partnership built on mutual respect and admiration. If you aren't willingly committed to providing your horse with the very best, you can't expect them to willingly give you their best in return. If you could ask your horse, what would he or she say about your relationship? Would you get a good report?

Does your horse know or feel how much you care?

Giving your horse your best goes beyond providing a comfortable stall and good feed; it includes *always* treating them with the most respect you can whenever you're with them. "Going beyond" includes a few more things to remember:

Leave Your Problems Behind

Maybe you had a tough day, or need to vent your anger or let off some steam, but remember the barn is not the place to dwell on those feelings. It's crucial to know that your horse has feelings too, and can read you better than you can sometimes read yourself. Just as the mood of people around you can affect you, your mood can affect your horse. After all, a horse can read your intentions from across the barn! I've had days when I arrived at the barn with residuals of a bad situation from earlier in the day, got my brushes out, and found myself brushing my horse so roughly that she had to move away from me. Our horse time can be one of our greatest opportunities to "be in the moment". If you're aware enough, the time can be used to completely change your day, enhance your outlook, and enrich your life.

Have Clear Intentions for Your Ride

When you arrive at the barn, it may be the end of your workday, but it's the beginning of your horse's day. If you feel the need to enjoy some leisure time, let your horse relax and just spend time together. It's not fair to expect your horse to focus if you're distracted. Your horse needs clear direction. This means giving your full attention when you ride and providing consistent, clear guidance on exactly what you want from them. There's a time for socializing and a time for focusing on your horse, and the two don't usually mix well. If your concentration is frequently being interrupted by conversations or the activities of others, it's unreasonable to expect your horse to maintain their concentration and return to the task at hand. It's also important to remember just how intuitively connected your horse may be to your thoughts. Disjointed patterns between focused time and casual time are frustrating for a horse. If the events of your day have left you physically or mentally fatigued, your horse will pick up on your de-motivated state and respond accordingly. Without positive input from you, don't expect a positive result. Even if it may have been your intention to work on a particular element of your riding in that session, if you're not focused, why would you expect your horse to be? Try to be flexible in your approach to riding and adjust your plans when necessary to best suit your mood *and* your horse's mood on any given day.

Rider Fitness – A Big Deal!

Not only does your day-to-day physical or mental state affect the horse in *every* aspect of the ride, *every* time you ride, so does your overall level of general fitness. No matter how well conditioned your horse is, if *you're* out of condition, you're simply making *their* work harder. As explained by author Linda Purves, in her book, *Horse and Rider Fitness – The essential guide for all riders*: "By increasing your fitness for riding, you will not only be benefiting yourself, but also your horse. You will be better placed to help rather than hinder when in the saddle, and you will be far better prepared to cope with the physical demands … without danger of injury to either party."

Getting in better shape may include going on a diet and losing a few pounds, but rider fitness isn't necessarily about embarking on a marathon-training program, it's about becoming a "light" rider. Taking steps to improve your balance, coordination, mobility and flexibility in the saddle is more important for your horse than how much you weigh. A 90-pound marathon runner who trains in the gym five days a week but is new to riding could effectively be heavier in the saddle than a 190-pound experienced rider who has never attended a gym. Maintaining a good level of general fitness is essential in terms of boosting your overall physical and mental health, particularly for horseback riding. The more in tune you are with your own body, the greater your ability to tune in to your horse's body. The more fit you are, the more physical and mental energy you have in the saddle. This not only lightens the load on your horse, it also allows you to continue to grow in terms of improving your riding skills.

Most people are right-handed or right-sided, but we shouldn't just ride that way by default. Neither should left-handed people. If we expect our horse to be balanced both ways, we should be too.

We usually write with one hand, brush our teeth with one hand, serve a volley with one hand, etc. It's our duty as riders to be as equally balanced as we ask our horses to be. This means we should work our weaker side twice as much as our stronger side. Try saddling your horse from the right side instead of the left and see what I mean. If we don't take our own bodies seriously, we will forever ride imbalanced and blame it on our horses. There are a lot of good books on rider fitness and I urge you to investigate some of them for yourself, not only to increase your own awareness, but also to hopefully inspire you to be a "better ride" for your horse.

Choosing a Mentor

In any sport, no one gets to the top of their game alone; horseback riding is no different. Athletes who make it into their sport's Hall of Fame usually credit a long list of people for helping them get to where they are. At least one coach or mentor will most likely be responsible for much of someone's final progress toward a goal. You don't need to be aiming for the Olympics to need the assistance of a mentor. An appropriately skilled individual who understands both you and your horse can be a benefit as an experienced pair of "eyes on the ground" to monitor your riding skills. Whatever your goals are as a rider, or whatever level of riding you're aiming to achieve, a mentor can provide guidance, advice, support, inspiration, and motivation to be your best.

Ultimately, your heart and your mentor's heart must line up.

BEFORE THE CROP COMES OUT...KEY POINT TO CONSIDER NUMBER 8

KNOW WHO YOU ARE AS A RIDER.

Follow Your Heart

Try answering the following questions with total honesty:

- Do you look forward with excitement to your training sessions?
- Does your instructor support and encourage you with a positive attitude when learning new ideas?
- Are you most always clear about what has been learned or gained in a session?
- Do you feel safe in your sessions?
- Do you enjoy your trainer or instructor?
- Do you feel comfortable about doing things that are asked of you?
- Are you making adequate progress in relation to others in similar training or riding programs?
- Have you considered expanding your knowledge or skills? Is your trainer supportive of other sources of learning, including other trainers?

If your answers are "yes", this is a good sign that your heart is lined up with your instructor or trainer's heart and you're learning with your complete HEART and SOUL. If your answers cause you to pause and think, maybe a change is in order.

Your choice of instructor or trainer may be limited by the availability of trainers or riding instructors at your ranch or in your area. Maybe someone was referred to you. In the U.S., there's no license requirement for horse trainers or riding instructors. *Anybody* can claim to be an expert, whether they've had any experience or not. It's amazing how many of us will immediately assume that one is an expert trainer or instructor just because they say so. For example, what does "riding since the age of six" *really* tell you? Having a business card or website doesn't make someone qualified. Even teaching credentials don't demonstrate *real* experience or intuition. An unpleasant experience with an amateur instructor can permanently ruin your enthusiasm, not to mention your pocketbook. Horse owners can spend thousands of dollars over time on lessons or training. For all these reasons and more, it's in your best interest to make the most educated decision possible so that you can get the best possible results. Take the time to interview and observe a prospective trainer or instructor. Watch them ride; watch a number of lessons or sessions. What do you notice from the sidelines? Try to get a *feel* for whether their heart lines up with your own.

It's also important to note that there can be a distinct difference between a riding instructor and a horse trainer, although the word trainer is often used interchangeably.

Instructor = communication is focused primarily on the rider so any communication made with the horse is through the rider.

Trainer = communication is focused primarily on teaching the horse through the trainer. Rider may be secondary.

Finding an individual with the skills to understand and communicate clearly with both the rider and the horse can be difficult. Those who can manage this task are very valuable. It's also good to know that your first instructor or trainer may or may not work out. The best you can do in that situation is to follow your instincts. The individual in question may have come highly recommended, but the right mentor for *you* is one who has the appropriate education and experience needed to help *you* progress in your riding and achieves *your* goals and ambitions with your horse. Don't forget that as we progress, so will our needs. You might come across someone that can take you further than your current trainer or instructor. Always be open to growth, and learn from as many sources as you can.

I should mention here that unfortunately, some riders might not be well matched to their horse. This can be hard to see, and even more difficult to accept, but a good instructor/trainer should be able to help you determine this with care, truth and respect.

The most important qualifications your mentor must have are an *intuitive* understanding of you as a rider, an intuitive understanding of what your horse needs, and how to best communicate with you both.

My Wish for Every Horse and Rider

All in all, it's been my desire to share my own learning experiences in the hope that you find them helpful. If my experiences resonate with you, or you recognize some of my challenges in your own situation with your own horse, I urge you to look further into the needs of your horse, rather than just at the behavior they may display in an effort to communicate those needs. Maybe you'll be able to enjoy your horse more, and enjoy your role as a caretaker and partner with your equine friend. My hope is that you'll realize, *Before the 'Crop' Comes Out*, that your horse's "bad behavior" isn't necessarily the result of your horse being obstinate; it may instead be the result of your horse being uncomfortable or in pain. Your horse might simply need more understanding, attention or love. I believe that approaching a horse with grace can teach us to better understand their "heart and soul." The journey into the amazing world of understanding and loving a horse can show us a true reflection of the love we have for ourselves and for others… after all, we all need a little grace.

Wrapping It Up

The 8 Essentials to Consider Before Disciplining Your Horse

1 **Does your horse have sound legs and correct shoes?**

   Check regularly for early warning signs of potential lameness. Pay attention to your horse's standing surface. Make allowances for new or varied riding surfaces. Check your horse's feet for correct angles and balance. Consult with a good farrier and be prepared to ask the right questions.

2 **Does your horse have muscle stress or back problems?**

   Take steps to alleviate stress in your horse's body. Check for signs of hidden back pain, and for proper spine alignment before expecting your horse to perform. Have an equine chiropractor on your team. Check your horses' back on a regular basis.

3 **Does your saddle fit?**

   Check your saddle(s) for basic fit and get a professional fit analysis. Be sure that your saddles fit, both horse and rider. If not, research what to do and how to look for a correctly fitted saddle.

4 **Are you using an appropriate, correctly fitting bit?**

   Know your bit (purpose and function). Examine your horse's mouth to determine if your bits fit. Use a bit that's appropriate for your horse's age and level of training, and for you as a rider. Consider a custom bit, if needed.

5 **Is your horse underfed or overfed, or in need of dental work?**

   Know your horse's feeding times. Feed regularly and often. Know what's in their diet and if they're getting the correct food. Make sure your horse gets the proper amount of food, and adjust if necessary. Use the appropriate food for your horse's age and level of activity. Routinely have your horse's teeth floated, and check for dental issues.

6 **Is your horse out of shape?**

   Warm up and stretch your horse. Know your horse's limits. Time their workouts. Have a conditioning plan. Cross train. Notice if, or when your horse is bored. Take the time to cool-down. Be flexible in your approach.

7 **Do you have a complete, personal horse care routine?**

   Take time to groom thoroughly. Check the legs, feet and joints each day for small changes in temperature or swelling. Have a well-organized grooming kit. Try to get your horse out of their stall daily. Provide enough bedding for them to be comfortable. Make sure the stall is kept clean. Keep a health care calendar.

8. **Do you know who you are as a rider?**

   Honestly assess your commitment to riding. Ask yourself what your horse might say if he or she was to give you a review. Set clear intentions for your rides. Examine *your* level of fitness. Be in balance with your horse. Ask yourself if you enjoy your riding or training sessions. Interview a prospective trainer or instructor and observe them working with others. Be sure your trainer or instructor's attitude and instinct lines up with yours.

   I hope you find inspiration in this and have a long life of
   Healthy **E**njoyment **A**nd **R**espectful **T**eamwork in a **S**pirit **O**f **U**nderstanding and **L**ove.
   The **HEART** and **SOUL** of horse ownership.

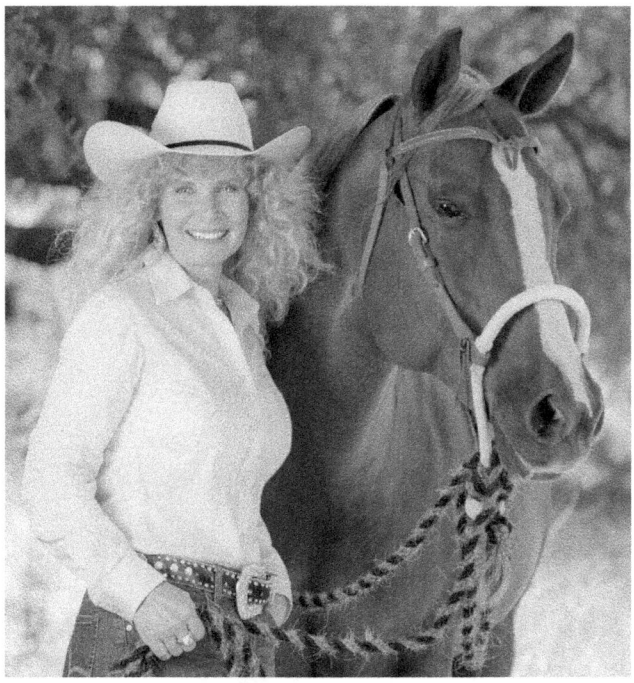

Author, Sandi Bell, with her horse Grace.

Resources

American Veterinarian Chiropractic Association
www.animalchiropractic.org

The Original Bit Fit Equine Mouth Measurement Tool
theoriginalbitfit.com

Equestrian Impressions
Equestrianimpressions.com

Equine Studies Institute
www.equinestudiesinstitute.com

Equinology
www.equinology.com

Farnam –Excalibur Sheath Cleaner for Horses
www.farnam.com

JC Dill Photography
portfolio.jcdill.com

The Masterson Method
www.mastersonmethod.com

Myler Bits USA
www.mylerbitsusa.com

Steel Saddle Tree LLC
www.equi-flex.com

Bibliography

Billington, Galadriel, *Saddle Fitting Essentials for the horse lover*, Lorien Press, Alachua County, FL, (2006)

Harman, Joyce, *The Western Horse's Pain-Free Back and Saddle-Fit Book*, Trafalgar Square, North Pomfret, VT (2008)

Harman, Joyce, *The Horse's Pain-Free Back and Saddle-Fit Book*, Trafalgar Square, North Pomfret, VT (2004)

Hill, Cherry, *How To Think Like a Horse*, Storey Publishing, North Adams, MA (2006)

Krolick, David, *Shoeing Right*, Breakthrough Publishing, Ossining, New York, NY (1991)

Meagher, Jack, *Beating Muscle Injuries for Horses*, Hamilton Horse Associates, Hamilton, MA (1985)

Myler, Dale, Ron & Bob, *The Level Best for Your Horse: the Myler Bitting System*, Toklat Originals, Inc., Lake Oswego, OR (2010)

Purves, Linda, *Horse and Rider Fitness: The essential guide for all riders*, Kenilworth Press, Shrewsbury, Shropshire, UK (2006)

Rashid, Mark, *Whole Heart, Whole Horse*, Sky Horse Publishing, New York, NY (2009)

Wyche, Sara, *Understanding The Horse's Back*, The Crowood Press, Ramsbury, Marlborough, Wiltshire, Great Britain (2001)

Wyche, Sara, *Understanding The Horse's Legs*, The Crowood Press, Ramsbury, Marlborough, Wiltshire, Great Britain (2000)

Notes

www.ingramcontent.com/pod-product-compliance
Lightning Source LLC
Chambersburg PA
CBHW081355040426
42451CB00017B/3463